Latin American Societies

Current Challenges in Social Sciences

This series aims at presenting to the international community original contributions by scholars working on Latin America. Such contributions will address the challenges that Latin American societies currently face as well as the ways they deal with these challenges. The series will be methodologically agnostic, that is: it welcomes case studies, small-N comparative studies or studies covering the whole region, as well as studies using qualitative or quantitative data (or a mix of both), as long as they are empirically rigorous and based on high-quality research. Besides exploring Latin American challenges, the series attempts to provide concepts, findings and theories that may shed light on other regions. The series will focus on five axes of challenges:

1) Social, Public and Environmental Policies

The first set of challenges revolves around the agenda setting in public and social policies in Latin America. This may include several topics like: redistribution policies, social mobility, marginalization. Another key item to be included deals with sources and consequences of environmental change – especially human-related change. These consequences threaten not only Latin American's material reproduction (e. g. by threatening water and food sources) but also deeply ingrained cultural practices and lifestyles. This section will, therefore, include proposals on environmental policies and matters. We welcome studies on a wide array of social, public and environmental policy making, implementation and effects.

2) Crime, Security and Violence

The second set of challenges stem from the persistence of violence and insecurity among Latin Americans, which consistently rank crime and insecurity at the top of their biggest problems. Crime organizations – from youth gangs to drug cartels – have grown and became more professionalized, displacing state forces in considerable chunks of national territories and, in some cases, penetrating the political class through illegal campaign funding and bribes. To this we should add, in some countries of the region, the persistence of armed insurgents fighting against governmental forces and paramilitaries, therefore creating cross-fires that threaten the lives of civilians. We welcome studies on a wide array of security and violence related issues.

3) Collective Action

A third theme has to do with how collective actors – social movements, civil society organizations, and quasi-organized groups – deal with issues that affect them. We welcome studies on a wide array of collective actors working on different issues, with different tactics, and diverse ideological stances.

4) Migrations

Political, economic, and environmental crises, as well as promises of better opportunities in other lands, have encouraged Latin Americans to migrate within their national borders or beyond them. While during the 1970s Latin Americans often migrated to other regions, nowadays national crises encourage them to seek other destinations in more nearby countries. We welcome studies on a wide array of topics and diverse theoretical perspectives.

5) Political Inclusion and Quality of Democracy

Dealing with social and ethnic minorities constitutes one of the most recurrent and unresolved challenges for the Latin American democracies. This topic includes the representation of the minorities, but includes also the study of the socio-political elites. We also welcome other studies on a wide array of issues regarding inclusion and quality of democracy in the region.

Both solicited and unsolicited proposals will be considered for publication in the series.

Isamu Okada
Editor

COVID-19 and State Capacity in Latin America

Comparative Perspectives on Responses to the Pandemic

Springer

Editor
Isamu Okada
Graduate School of International Development
Nagoya University
Nagoya, Japan

ISSN 2730-5538 ISSN 2730-5546 (electronic)
Latin American Societies
ISBN 978-3-032-15571-9 ISBN 978-3-032-15572-6 (eBook)
https://doi.org/10.1007/978-3-032-15572-6

This work was supported by Japan Society for the Promotion of Science (20KK0024).

This Springer imprint is published by the registered company Springer Nature Switzerland AG
The registered company address is: Gewerbestrasse 11, 6330 Cham, Switzerland

Preface

COVID-19 has apparently become a past event in people's minds. Latin American countries are rife with political and economic problems that preoccupy people more than the pandemic as early as the end of 2020, according to Latinobarometro. Yet, the fact that there are too many events to worry about in life doesn't mean each problem is minor. The COVID-19 pandemic remains in the memory of many Latin American people, who often lost their families or friends due to the infection. Medical professionals lament weak preparations and scarce resources, especially at the onset, and people recall tragedies even a couple of years after the situation has normalized. This book could have been a battery of such narratives, which must also be moving and illustrative.

In mid-2020, when the onset of negative consequences unfolded, we launched this project and decided to focus on state capacity. We had previously studied diverse social issues in Latin America that were left unsolved due to weak state capacity and had no doubt that the pandemic would become a new page. Also, it was obvious that the pandemic, as a common challenge to countries worldwide, was a stress test that would reveal state capacity variation. Indeed, in 2020, weak state capacity and the accelerated spread of the virus obliged many Latin American countries to introduce strict lockdowns, notwithstanding the severe consequences that followed.

Then, several months were spent articulating our theoretical framework. State capacity, widely discussed in the Introduction, is conceptual luggage that is uneasy to pin down in a rapidly unfolding crisis. A foggy mixture of various factors often obfuscates what should be regarded as a capacity limitation and what is not. Disentangling state capacity and its limitations from policymakers' decisions later became the foundation of our argument. Some of us worked heavily on acquiring new data and methodologies. We hope that, in the end, the chapters in our collection disclose insightful aspects of state capacity limitations and collectively tell a story that is theoretically meaningful.

Besides theoretical contributions, the pandemic must be a lesson to inform what could be improved. Political actors come and go as time passes, but state capacity remains the baseline for those responsible for future challenges. It might be possible to constrain arbitrary decisions by political leaders and enhance constructive leadership. Yet, any leaders without state capacity cannot effectively implement their choices and must play their roles with limited options, scope, and impact. Political decisions without proper state capacity tend to become unclear, uninformed, and aspirational, if not erroneous. We hope our work becomes a cornerstone for academic society, policymakers, and civil society actors who ask for practical solutions.

This edited volume is a product of a multi-year collaboration. It is fully supported by JSPS KAKENHI 20KK0024 for funding all activities related to this project, including the book processing charge for open access. Takahiro, Hirokazu, and Shuichiro have been core members of this grant project from the beginning, providing careful and always helpful comments in the entire process.

The fund's generous support also enabled international collaborations, which could otherwise have been impossible. A panel titled "State Capacity and COVID-19 in Latin America," which was held at the conference of the International Political Science Association in Buenos Aires on July 19, 2023, gave us the first chance to introduce this project to a global community, particularly Latin American academia. Many people in the panel discussion, especially Marcus Andres Mello from the Federal University of Pernambuco, Brazil, commented critically and productively. On that occasion, Cecilia and Gabriela joined our team with a paper that later evolved as a chapter of this edited volume. Jennifer Cyr from the Universidad Torquato di Tella also supported our project at this early instance.

In March 2024, we organized an international workshop in Mexico City hosted by Colegio de Mexico in collaboration with the University of Tokyo. Ilan was an excellent host there, convoking his colleagues, Juan José Ramírez, Juan Cruz Olmeda, and Mariano Sánchez-Talanquer, who brought their works to the discussion among other chapter contributors. Although their papers finally found other homes, the intensive discussion polished other papers that remained in this collective endeavor. Matias and Fiorella traveled to this event with a paper that eventually became a chapter.

Later, Takahiro and Isamu had an opportunity to receive constructive suggestions at a QCA workshop at Waseda University on September 3, 2024, which was also supported by JSPS KAKENHI 23K17283. Sho Niikawa, Airo Hino, Andreas Corcaci, and Marisa Kellam, among others, commented on our two papers, improving the application of qualitative comparative analysis.

In the editing process, two anonymous reviewers provided critical and constructive suggestions that sharpened our argument and content. Melina Neophytou and Sultane Mussa helped with careful checks on the first and second drafts. My colleagues, supported and provided advice in editing. Last but not least, the Springer editing team supplied effective support. Many thanks to everyone.

Nagoya, Aichi, Japan Isamu Okada

Contents

Contributors

Matías Bianchi is the founder and director of Asuntos del Sur, a think-do tank focused on political innovations for improving democracies in the Global South. He received PhD in Political Science from Sciences Po, MSc from the University of Oxford, an MPA from Sciences Po, and a BA from the University of Buenos Aires. He has worked for the Latin American Program of the Woodrow Wilson Center, the UNDP, the Government of Argentina, and the Development Center of the OECD and also led the Instituto Federal de Gobierno. He lectures at the University of Arizona (USA) and at DiTella (Argentina). His areas of research include politics in the digital age, democratic governance, and public innovation. He is co-editing a forthcoming book on collaborative governance (Fondo de Cultura Económica).

Ilán Bizberg is a professor-researcher at the Centro de Estudios Internacionales, El Colegio de México. He holds a PhD in Social Sciences from the École des Hautes Études en Sciences Sociales. He has been a visiting professor or researcher at Sciences Po, Paris and Poitiers, at the University of Paris III, at the EHESS, at the Fondation Maison des Sciences de l'Homme, at the CNRS-CREDAL, at the LAI of the Freie Universität Berlin, at the University of Bochum, and at the Woodrow Wilson Center, Washington. His most recent books are *Diversity of Capitalisms in Latin America*, Palgrave, Macmillan, 2019 and *Four Worlds of the Welfare State in Latin America*, Palgrave-Macmillan, 2024. In 2020, he received the Alexander von Humboldt Foundation Research Prize.

Gabriela Bortz is an assistant professor at the Research Center for Transformation, Economics & Business School, Universidad Nacional de San Martín (CENIT-EEyN-UNSAM/CONICET, Argentina) and Associate Professor of Science, Technology, and Society (STS) at Universidad Nacional de Hurlingham. A political scientist with an MA and Ph.D. in Science, Technology, and Innovation Policy and Politics, she was a Fulbright Fellow at the Harvard Program on Science, Technology and Society (2021) and Brocher Foundation Fellow (2024). Her research explores STI policies, socio-technical imaginaries, and biotechnology governance for development in Latin America. She received several awards, including the Marcel Roche Award for Young STS Scholars (ESOCITE, 2024) and Best Policy Research (SAAP, 2017).

Florencia Coda is a political scientist and professor at the Universidad Torcuato Di Tella's Political Science Department. Her research focuses on gender equity, governance, and public innovation in Latin America. She has extensive experience managing and coordinating research projects across Latin America and the Caribbean, specializing in governance and the strategic development of alliances with NGOs, governments, and the private sector. She co-authored a policy brief for the T20 on vaccine governance for the Global South and actively collaborates with civil society organizations on initiatives that promote women's leadership and economic empowerment. Her work bridges academia and policy, fostering collaborative solutions for inclusive and sustainable development.

Hirokazu Kikuchi is a senior research fellow at the Area Studies Center at the Institute of Developing Economies (IDE-JETRO), Chiba, Japan. He earned his doctoral degree in political science from the University of Pittsburgh. His research focuses on legislative politics, executive-legislative relations, electoral systems, voting behavior, and civil society organizations with a regional emphasis on Latin America. His work has appeared in *Frontiers in Psychology*, *Issues and Studies*, *Journal of Politics in Latin America*, and *Journal of Behavioral Public Administration*. He is the author of *Presidents versus Federalism in the National Legislative Process: The Argentine Senate in Comparative Perspective* (Palgrave Macmillan, 2018).

Shuichiro Masukata is an associate professor in the Faculty of Law at Keio University, Japan. Before his current position, he was a lecturer in the Department of Spanish and Portuguese at Kanda University of International Studies and an associate professor at the Graduate School of Global Studies at Tokyo University of Foreign Studies, Japan. He specializes in international relations and Brazilian politics. He has written chapters in *Partnership for a Change: Toward a Framework of Brazil-Japan Cooperation*, edited by N. Hamaguchi and D. Ramos, Springer (2022), and *Non-Western Nations and the Liberal International Order: Responses to the Backlash against the Global Spread of Liberalism, edited by* H. Kusano and H. Katsumata, Routledge (2023).

Takahiro Miyachi is a professor of comparative politics at the Graduate School of Arts and Sciences, The University of Tokyo. His research focuses on Latin American politics, particularly political participation. He has conducted extensive fieldwork in Bolivia and Ecuador and has been a visiting researcher at Universidad Mayor de San Andrés and FLACSO Ecuador. His work is widely published in Spanish, appearing in *Decursos* (Bolivia), *De Política* (Mexico), *Ecuador Debate*, and various edited volumes in Latin America. He has also collaborated on international research projects examining development governance, public policies related to Indigenous rights, and Japan–Latin America relations from a comparative perspective.

Isamu Okada is a political scientist and a professor at the Graduate School of International Development, Nagoya University. Before his current position, he worked at the Japanese Embassy in the Plurinational State of Bolivia and as a Postdoctoral Research Fellow at the Japan Society for Promotion of Science. His research interest ranges from resource governance, political participation, Latin American politics, and, most recently, the social impacts of COVID-19. His academic works have been published in *World Development*, *the Journal of Behavioral Public Administration*, *Frontiers in Psychology*, and *Humanities and Social Sciences Communications*. He has ample fieldwork experience in Bolivia, Peru, and other Latin American countries.

Cecilia Sanmartin has a degree in biotechnology (Universidad Nacional de Quilmes, Argentina) and a master's degree in Science, Technology and Society (Universidad Nacional de Quilmes, Argentina). She is currently pursuing a PhD in Economics of Innovation (CENIT-EEyN-Universidad Nacional de San Martin). She specializes in the analysis of the development and production of vaccines in Argentina from a theoretical triangulation between the sociology of technology and the sociology of expectations. She has various publications that seek to analyze the co-production between situated symbolic elements (imaginaries and visions of what is good and desirable) and scientific-technological dynamics.

Sofia Santamarina holds a degree in Political Science from the University of Buenos Aires (Argentina), a Master's in Human Rights and Democratization in Latin America and the Caribbean from the National University of San Martín (Argentina), and is currently pursuing a Master's in Political Science at the Torcuato Di Tella University (Argentina). She works as an advisor at the Political Rights Observatory of the Ombudsperson's Office of Buenos Aires, as a project assistant at the think-to-do tank Asuntos del Sur, as a university lecturer, and as an independent consultant. She is a member of the Red de Politólogas #NoSinMujeres. Her research focuses on political participation, electoral governance, and big data analysis.

Chapter 1
Introduction: Revisiting State Capacity on the COVID-19 Pandemic

Isamu Okada

1.1 Introduction

The COVID-19 pandemic has hit the Latin American region the hardest. As of October 2023, more than 80 million people were reported infected, and more than 1.7 million lost their lives.[1] The tremendous cost occurred despite strict confinement measures deployed in several countries, Argentina and Peru in particular, provoking suspicions about the effectiveness of preventive and containment measures. Questions revolved around the factors explaining uneven practices and outcomes in non-pharmaceutical interventions (NPI) and their societal appraisal (Alicea-Planas et al., 2021; Boruchowicz & Lopez Boo, 2022; Love & Smith, 2021).

Among myriad debates surrounding this conundrum, this book focuses on state capacity, which many scholars suggest as one of the key explanans for the COVID-19 outcomes worldwide (Aydın-Düzgit et al., 2023; Capano et al., 2020; Greer et al. 2020; Moisio, 2020). This attention is intuitively logical. Although the coronavirus started spreading from China, strong states in East Asia were the most successful in containing the damage during the early years (Yan et al., 2020). Not only China but also Taiwan, Hong Kong, South Korea, Singapore, and Japan were equipped with "institutional infrastructure and capacity before the COVID-19 pandemic arrived at their doorsteps" (An & Tang, 2020: 791). Conversely, South America, where state

[1] The Johns Hopkins Coronavirus Resource Center, https://coronavirus.jhu.edu/region, Accessed June 2022.

I. Okada (✉)
Nagoya University, Nagoya, Japan
e-mail: okada.isamu.w8@f.mail.nagoya-u.ac.jp

I. Okada (ed.), *COVID-19 and State Capacity in Latin America*, Latin American Societies, https://doi.org/10.1007/978-3-032-15572-6_1

capacity was considered weak, recorded the highest number of infected cases and deaths[2] (Fig. 1.1).

At the global level, cross-national empirical studies argue that stronger state capacity coincided with attenuated COVID-19 deaths and the augmented effect of lockdown measures (Alfano & Ercolano, 2022; Bosancianu et al., 2020; Serikbayeva et al., 2021). Cross-national and cross-subnational studies on Latin America in the early months of the corona pandemic (González-Bustamante, 2021; Schaefer et al., 2020) confirmed that the health sector capacities shaped divergent responses by the governments, urging those with low capacity to take quicker and more severe lockdowns in the early months.

Although some studies have suggested the nexus between state capacity and the effective responses to the COVID-19 pandemic, this linkage remains opaque. Table 1.1 summarizes some statistics related to COVID-19 and state capacity among Latin American countries. Looking at the imbalance between confirmed cases and deaths—what is usually called case fatality rates—some countries like Peru, Mexico, and Ecuador outpaced others. These countries have relatively smaller volumes of hospital beds and health expenditure available for the population size. Argentina, Chile, Panama, and Uruguay, better equipped with health infrastructures, scored better in the health performance.

However, this basic snapshot also leaves suspicions. Confirmed cases are often conditioned by testing capacity to accurately diagnose the infection of coronavirus, which may cause underreporting. Excess mortality in Table 1.1 reports some cases, like Bolivia, potentially biased by this limitation. Also, we notice outliers, such as the Dominican Republic, which are weak in health infrastructures but effective in mitigating the health impact.

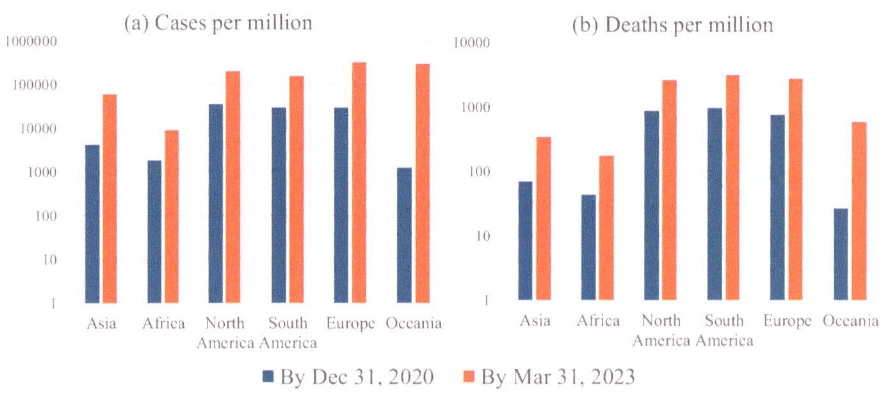

Fig. 1.1 Cases and deaths per million by region. Source: Our World in Data COVID-19 dataset

[2] State capacity is, of course, not the only explanatory factor. This is reflected in Fig. 1.1 where Africa and Oceania scored smaller numbers of cases and deaths, contradictory to the intuition derived from state capacity levels.

Table 1.1 Descriptive statistics related to COVID-19 and state capacity for Latin American countries

	Cumulative cases per million, by July 20, 2025	Confirmed deaths per million, by July 20, 2025	Deaths/ cases	Excess mortality per million, by Feb 28, 2022	Hospital beds per 10,000, latest before 2020	Health expenditure per capita, 2019	Government effectiveness, 2019
Peru	135,402.9	6603.6	4.88%	5750	15.91	366.2	46.7
Mexico	59,311.0	2604.5	4.39%	5488	9.8	515.4	39.0
Ecuador	60,613.8	2023.1	3.34%	4071	13.93	485.4	37.6
Paraguay	108,833.7	2940.7	2.70%	4025	8.28	391.9	32.4
Honduras	45,201.5	1062.1	2.35%	NA	6.43	192	30.5
Colombia	123,692.0	2759.7	2.23%	3483	17.1	470.3	53.8
El Salvador	32,168.8	673.5	2.09%	NA	11.99	362.3	34.3
Brazil	179,525.3	3342.7	1.86%	3473	20.87	684.2	41.9
Bolivia	100,369.5	1853.8	1.85%	5225	12.93	234.7	21.9
Guatemala	70,226.3	1132.1	1.61%	2675	4.41	293.6	26.2
Nicaragua	2436.3	36.4	1.49%	2639	9.3	165.4	22.9
Argentina	222,729.5	2880.2	1.29%	3577	49.92	911.3	48.1
Chile	276,692.8	3215.5	1.16%	2334	20.6	1315.8	77.6
Venezuela	19,591.8	207.6	1.06%	NA	8.71	114.6	4.3
Panama	237,565.5	1999.4	0.84%	NA	22.54	1294.4	57.6
Costa Rica	243,798.8	1847.0	0.76%	1285	11	920.1	66.2
Uruguay	307,536.8	2269.3	0.74%	1710	24.25	1562.6	73.3
Dominican Rep	58,865.8	390.4	0.66%	938	15.56	329.3	38.1

Source: Author's own calculations based on Our World in Data COVID-19 dataset, World Development Indicators, and Worldwide Governance Indicators

Moreover, we acknowledge that the current index of state capacity does not capture the importance of state capacity matters to the COVID-19 responses from the cross-country comparison in Table 1.1. A frequently used state capacity proxy, Government Effectiveness in the Worldwide Governance Indicators of the World Bank, has weak explanatory power on the health outcomes.[3] This does not automatically mean that state capacity does not matter; rather, the Government Effectiveness index is possibly too generic to capture what and how state capacity matters in the pandemic.

Furthermore, this snapshot does not tell what governments could or could not do at critical moments, like at the onset of the pandemic. The mechanism that channels state capacity to measures is a dynamic process that involves interactions among multiple factors. In the global crisis unfolding, the states elaborated measures, learned from others, and implemented solutions with any available resources in

[3] Pierson's correlation index is 0.319 with 0.197 as the p-value.

cooperation within and beyond the state apparatus. Hence, state capacity also means the policy coordination, implementation, and communicational acts that make policies effective.

Overall, our understanding of state capacity and how it matters to the pandemic has been very limited. As discussed later in this chapter, while much of the previous literature focused on political choices and societal structures, the state capacity perspective has received scant attention.

Latin America provides a useful set of cases and episodes for addressing this critical gap for several reasons. The region recorded the highest suffering from the COVID-19 pandemic compared to other regions in the world (see Fig. 1.1). This fact alone demands a closer look at the regional experience. Besides, rich debates from the regional contexts have created a good level of conceptual precision regarding state capacity and also confirmed structural variations among regional countries over history. This provides an analytical advantage of the regional focus. Last, but not least, deeper dives into the regional experience provide comparative lessons. Being a common challenge to all countries in the world, the global pandemic "presents a rare naturally occurring experiment" (Liu & Geva-May, 2021, 132). We entrust that a comparative view of the Latin American countries, as the most comparable set, provides nuanced lessons that a single-country study or global comparison may not achieve.

1.2 Questions of This Book

This book's main objective is to fill the critical void regarding the relationship between state capacity in the COVID pandemic. Our contestations are threefold.

First, state capacity as an explanatory factor for the pandemic outcomes has so far received surprisingly little attention in Latin America, despite the fact that the concept has been a subject of long debate in the region. Comparative studies in the last decade accumulated rich debates on the origins and outcomes of divergent state capacity as well as the conceptualization and empirical measurements (Centeno et al., 2017; Kurtz, 2013; Luna & Soifer, 2017; Saylor, 2014; Soifer, 2008, 2015). At the same time, the causes and consequences of uneven state capacity have been a popular debate in social welfare provision at both national and subnational levels (Niedzwiecki, 2018; Segura-Ubiergo, 2007).

Latin American countries are similar in historical backgrounds from colonial heritage but rich in diversity regarding federal and unitary states, pre-pandemic institutional strengths, and the expansion of welfare regimes (Bizberg, 2024; Mahoney, 2010). Some of the remarkable characteristics, such as strong presidencies and welfare systems, are already studied in relation to the pandemic (Blofield et al., 2023; Fernandez & Machado, 2021). Still, how best the states responded to the pandemic and where the capacity limitations lie has received scant attention.

Second, as recent studies suggest (Brinks et al., 2020; Centeno et al., 2017; Helmke & Levitsky, 2004; Holland, 2017), state strengths and weaknesses are not the end of the analysis. Weak policy implementation at the national level may derive not only from the limited state capacity of the national states but also from unsmooth or uncooperative coordination between the national and subnational governments and between the state and societal actors. Even if the state or national government cannot react sufficiently to life risks, responses may emerge from subnational governments and civil society organizations to fill the capacity gap.

In this vein, collaborative governance (Cyr et al., 2021) sheds light on collaborations, or lack thereof, among various actors. Subnational governments are responsible for health policy administrations in the federal states and other decentralized regimes. Societal actors, such as universities, businesses, and professional associations, can provide technical support, and those like labor unions, neighborhood associations, and caregiving organizations may help in the implementation process. Hence, various responses could emerge from the state and social actors, and multilevel governance in critical moments must be assessed for their potential to fill capacity limitations.

Third, state capacity as a concept must be closely revisited in light of the pandemic. The pandemic provides a unique opportunity to update the state capacity as a theoretical concept. The making and implementation of infection-preventive measures have relied on the capability of the state authority to deploy health infrastructure, provide timely and extensive health services, and mobilize policy tools to build desirable collective actions either by coercive or non-coercive means. Knowing what capacity limitations existed and how the states addressed them provides lessons to policymakers preparing for another health crisis in the future.

Among the few, the previous studies relied on the Government Effectiveness in Worldwide Governance Indicators (WGI) (Serikbayeva et al., 2021) and the Fragile State Index (FSI) (Gisselquist & Vaccaro, 2023). While these indicators help to capture general trends, they hardly approach what specific capacity matters within the health sector. How effective were the states in imposing stringent lockdowns and nudging people to change their behavior? How much was their legibility, like scaling up their capacity to supply PCR kits and implement diagnoses? What were the bottlenecks in other services, like drafting emergent orders and importing or inventing vaccines? Addressing those questions and improving state capacity measurements would be a meaningful lesson from the pandemic, which created a common stress check for regional countries.

To address these gaps, we revisit the state capacity concept and renew our understanding of the pandemic by assessing it through the state capacity lens. The following three research questions guide our discussion in this book.

- What do state strengths and weaknesses explain about the responses and outcomes to the COVID-19 pandemic?
- What solutions were practically available when state capacity was weak or limited?
- What does the COVID-19 pandemic update with the meaning of state capacity?

In the following sections, we clarify our definitions and standpoints. Section 1.3 sets our working definition of state capacity. Section 1.4 provides a brief overview of state capacity and state-building in Latin America. Section 1.5 explains how our focus on state capacity is related to other explanations in the extant COVID-19 studies. Section 1.6 revisits the cases of weak state capacity and introduces how collaboration among state and non-state actors may work complementarily. Section 1.7 discusses methodological remarks. Finally, Sect. 1.8 summarizes an overview of the chapters.

1.3 Defining State Capacity

What is state capacity? We define it as the ability of the state to effectively implement its decisions over society. Our definition is mostly aligned with canonical understandings (Berwick & Christia, 2018; Cingolani, 2013; Lindvall & Teorell, 2016). The classic definition of infrastructural power by Mann (1984: 189) takes "the capacity of the state to actually penetrate civil society, and to implement logistically political decisions throughout the realm." Many studies followed this and argued for state capacity relative to the implementation process.

State capacity is usually argued as issue-dependent and hardly represented by a single indicator. In other words, strong capacity in one policy area can coexist with weak capacity in other issue areas. Especially in the scope of this book, which takes the case of COVID-19, it is related to the capacities associated with health measures.

The conceptual discussion over state capacity has been long and rich (Kurtz & Schrank, 2007; Soifer, 2008; Soifer & vom Hau, 2008), often critical of concept stretching and measurement problems. We don't mean to propose here a single, solid, and universally justifiable conceptualization. Rather, following Vaccaro (2023), we attempt to clarify our working definition and conceptual boundaries and the potential misuse that we want to avoid. To this end, we highlight a few critical remarks on our definition to demarcate what is state capacity from what is not.

1.3.1 Capacity of the State

State capacity must be a *capacity*, not a political choice or the will of the state. This may sound axiomatic, but it is critical to avoid confusion. For instance, Weiss and Thurbon (2022) propose "salutary capacity," which is "the state's ability to correct and counteract the course of a national health emergency." While the meaning of this statement is a bit ambiguous, they argue that such capacity performed well or worse depending on political choices. Strictly speaking, we don't consider this an issue of state capacity since, in general, political choices are about the making of a decision, not its implementation. In essence, capacity matters when a political choice is implemented, not when the choice is made.

When we call it a capacity, it should be separated from its outcomes. At this point, previous scholars are critical of cross-national indicators drawn from expert surveys, which tend to be post hoc assessments in the view of observers, mixing capacity with outcomes (Kurtz & Schrank, 2007). This is troublesome since outcomes may occur for ad hoc reasons regardless of the capacity level. Substituting capacity for its outcomes is often a suboptimal measurement strategy when studies cannot afford the proper measurement, which is frequently observed in cross-national studies. For instance, Gisselquist and Vaccaro (2023) used child mortality, school enrolment, access to drinking water, and perceptions of the quality of the state's basic administrative functions as a proxy for "Capacity," and other outcome information for "Authority" and "Legitimacy." This measurement choice is inevitably suboptimal, although frequently observed across many studies to fill data accessibility limitations.

Also, state capacity must be *of the state*, which means strong states should retain a certain level of autonomy from non-state actors (Soifer & vom Hau, 2008). State capacity can wax and wane through the interaction of politicians with social groups that possess specific policy preferences (Geddes, 1996). In certain cases, the state and societal actors may interact closely to pursue a common goal, complementing each other in terms of policy implementation (Evans, 1995). Still, the state with a substantive level of autonomy from social groups is different from the one without such autonomy—the latter should be judged a weak state (Migdal, 1988). What kind of autonomy we expect and how best it can be measured is not an easy task. We address this point in the following subsection.

1.3.2 Capacity to Implement Decisions on Social Interactions

While the implementation might sound like enforcing a will at a certain moment, our conceptualization includes preparation, coordination, regulation, and any interventions to align collective and individual actions with the state's objectives. This is echoed by most studies and recent conceptualization literature, which suggests state capacity can be disaggregated into extractive, coercive, and administrative (Hanson & Sigman, 2021) or extractive, coordination, and compliance capacities (Berwick & Christia, 2018). Here, extractive capacity is related to tax collection, and coercive and compliance capacities refer to state authorities that may exercise physical use of violence. Administrative or coordination capacities refer to the state's organizational structures that help implementation.

Here, we consider state capacity in a broader sense of policy implementation, which involves the capacity to crystallize policy ideas into concrete policy designs at a program level. National policies need to be implemented at subnational levels, requiring an additional policymaking process to design policy details (Ramírez de la Cruz et al., 2020).

Can we distinguish the phase of implementation from political choice? It is relatively easier at some points than the others. In early state intervention, governments adopted standard non-pharmaceutical interventions, such as testing, contact tracing, social contact restrictions, mask-wearing and hand-washing suggestions, border controls, and soft or hard lockdowns, etc., similar to most other countries worldwide. In the process, designing policy details belongs to the sphere of implementation, i.e., a part of state capacity.[4] Although political maneuvers may happen in such policy-designing phases, like tightening or softening movement restrictions in favor of some businesses or other sectors, it still broadly falls into the implementation domain. Conversely, if a government does not adopt such textbook interventions but makes other decisions drastically different, like the case of "deniers" (Fernandez & Machado, 2021), it is a question of political choice.

When we say the crystallization of ideas is a part of the implementation process, we envisage that policy elaboration and cooperation depend on bureaucrats who coordinate collective actions with key stakeholders and the institutional structure they can mobilize (Berwick & Christia, 2018). For example, recruiting talent experts and key stakeholders in the policy elaboration phase can improve state capacity in a short time, although not always enduring.

Also, trust in the state institution bears an important dimension (Bargain & Aminjonov, 2020). No matter how meritocratically capable the state administrative body is, an untrusted state would miss citizens' support. Previous literature concurs that compliance with state measures is robustly contingent on the trust people bestow on the authority (Pagliaro et al., 2021; Sarracino et al., 2024). In our viewpoint, trust (and distrust) is a non-institutional dimension of state capacity that affects policy implementation and compliance. We come back to the discussion of trust in a later section.

1.3.3 A Long-Term Factor

State capacity is generally a long-term factor that stays resilient over time. It is built path-dependently in the sense that a political choice at a time invests resources for institution-making that shapes an underlying baseline for policy implementation in the future. In this sense, we deploy the institutionalist perspective. Unsurprisingly, an institutional apparatus created in the past can be used to implement policy goals that fall outside of the original scope (Mahoney & Thelen, 2010).

In this sense, what Blofield et al. (2023) call "policy legacies" can be considered a state capacity. According to their explanation, policy legacies include established technical systems for conditional cash distribution that have existed since before the pandemic. This can entail various things, from resource allocation to vested and possibly segmented interests, some of which are evidently related to the capacity for policy implementation. In this sense, their "state capacity" represented by Worldwide Governance Indicators seems to address a generic remainder uncovered by "past legacies." Along the same line, the vaccine coverage for other epidemic viruses in

[4] The list of non-pharmaceutical interventions was mostly homogenous (Rausis & Hoffmeyer-Zlotnik, 2021; Sebhatu et al., 2020).

the past can represent a mix of different things, such as past policy outcomes, vaccine supply capacity, and people's acceptance of vaccines. Such distinction is of high interest if we want to know what exactly matters in state institutions and what we should improve for future challenges.

Considering state capacity as a long-term factor does not exclude the chance that state capacity changes in the short run. As recent literature argues (Dargent et al., 2017; Luna & Soifer, 2017), we assume state capacity evolves over time and is not fixed and left unchanged since a time in history. Institutional reforms may direct state financial and human resources to different sectors, improving or undermining administrative capacity. Also, a collaborative relationship with societal actors may quickly build up an implementation network necessary to speed up physical material supply, such as test toolkits, oxygen tanks, and vaccines, in urgency. Still, the change is hardly an abrupt and big leap from the status quo.

1.4 State Capacity in Latin America: A Brief Overview

Scholars have coincided that the early state-building during colonialism from the fifteenth to the nineteenth century and the period thereafter produced long-lasting impacts on state capacity in the region. As the nations were inserted into the global and colonial trade system from an early time, state infrastructure developed with a very limited territorial reach, concentrating on major resource hubs and export-oriented ports (Mazzuca, 2021).

Cross-national divergence became notable from the early stage, also due to the colonial legacy. In some countries where conservative rulers and oligarchies persisted in the exploitative industries of mines and agricultural plantations, such as Bolivia, Ecuador, Peru, and some others in Central America, inclusive and merit-based governance had less chance (Kurtz, 2013; Mahoney, 2010). In contrast, liberal elites in colonial peripheries, such as Argentina, Chile, Costa Rica, and Uruguay, took more emancipatory policies toward peasants, incorporated them into the political system from the early stage, and built more inclusive and equitable political institutions (Kurtz, 2013). According to Mahoney (2003, 2010), this divergence among regional peers marked the trend that persisted over centuries in socioeconomic development.

State-building attempts in the post-independent era constituted another layer, mainly by the centralization of state power in some countries, like Brazil and Chile, compared to delegated rules by local caudillos in others (Soifer, 2015). In Brazil, as an exception in the entire region, the developmental state paradigm gained momentum throughout the twentieth century, particularly during the era of Getulio Vargas (1930–1945), but also continuously in the later military governments (Leão, 2019). It was purported to reorganize state-society relations from a fragmented, regionalist toward centralized corporatism and build a stronger state apparatus with state-led industrial programs (Kohli, 2004). A similar attempt at state power centralization vis-à-vis subnational elites unfolded in Chile during the post-independent period in the nineteenth century (Kurtz, 2013; Soifer, 2015).

State capacity has been a gradual and geographically complex process throughout the twentieth century. Developmental drives expanded the state's reach toward subnational peripheries, usually driven by the mixed logic of economic imperatives and political competition (Saylor, 2014). Eaton (2017) explains that subnational hinterlands were usually left behind in national state-building when their economic importance was marginal, the central government lacked institutional capacity, and multi-level political coalitions were absent. In contrast, the state's territorial expansion could happen if any of the elements were present.

Another source for strengthening the institutional capacity of the state is the technocratic administrative reforms that occurred under neoliberal governments and other centralized statist regimes. Chile demonstrated some sorts of technocratic state-building from the time before the Pinochet regime, which invested in basic education and professional training (Silva, 2008). In Peru and Brazil, some state capacity improvements took shape by isolating technocratic policymakers from political and societal pressures (Geddes, 1996; Wise, 2003). This technocratic isolation reinforced some state capacity dimensions, such as tax collection and macroeconomic management, but remained insufficient in expanding the territorial penetration of basic services, including health.

Where are Latin American countries in terms of state capacity? Figure 1.2 illustrates the level of state capacity according to the dataset created by Hanson and Sigman (2021), one of the recent attempts to synthesize various dimensions and propose an integrated measurement.[5] For the sake of readability, we focus only on South American countries here. Comparatively speaking, some countries in the Southern Cone, namely Argentina, Chile, and Uruguay, scored higher state capacity levels. Other previous colonial centers that have been more populated by indigenous populations, such as Bolivia, Peru, and Mexico, recorded relatively lower capacity levels. This empirical snapshot coincides with the path-dependent arguments in previous literature (Kurtz, 2013; Mahoney, 2010), and also with what alternative state capacity measurements by Luna and Soifer (2017) reported.

The analyses in the following chapters will be developed in the context and rich accumulation of literature regarding the state-building and state capacity discussion. However, we focus specifically on state capacity aspects related to the COVID-19 pandemic. Hence, it is not our intention to integrate various dimensions of state capacity into one.

[5] The index is a product of Bayesian latent variable analysis based on numerous indicators, largely grouped into extractive (tax collection), coercive, and administrative capacities.

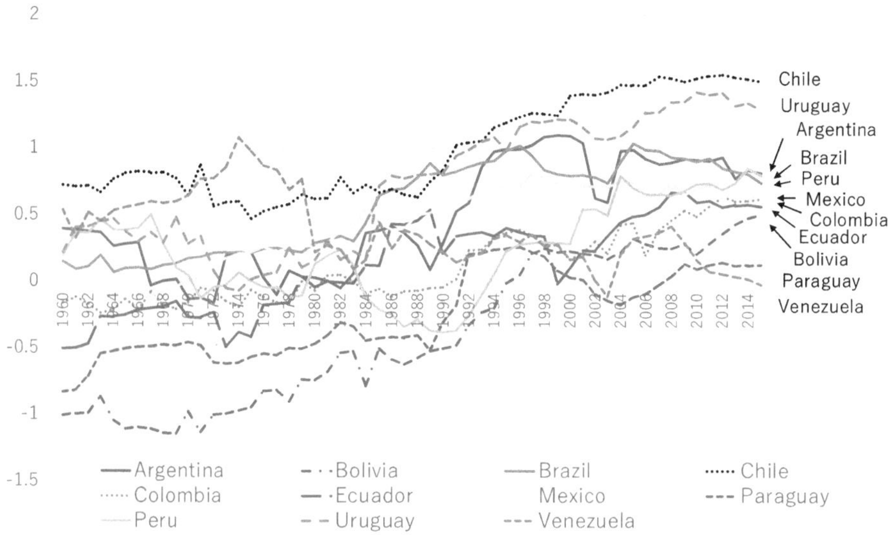

Fig. 1.2 State capacity score for South American countries and Mexico, 1960–2015. Source: Author's elaboration based on Hanson and Sigman (2021)

1.5 Relationship with Other COVID-19 Explanations

While we focus on state capacity in this book, there are plenty of works that talk about other factors explanatory for uneven reactions during the COVID-19 pandemic. We briefly review the two most influential ones: political agency and societal explanations. How is our state capacity discussion related to them?

1.5.1 Political Agency

Political decisions by national top executives have been argued as a major source of policy irregularities (Aydın-Düzgit et al., 2023; Boswell et al., 2021). It includes the character of the top leaders (Forster & Heinzel, 2021; Givens & Mistur, 2021) and the problem of miscommunication that failed to organize desirable collective action among people (García et al., 2020; Lasco, 2020). Also, the people's view toward the government, often relative to the partisanship, explains people's compliance across and within national territories[6] in Bolivia (Velasco-Guachalla et al., 2021), Brazil (Aruguete et al., 2021; Avritzer & Rennó, 2021; Batista Pereira & Nunes, 2021;

[6] Trust and partisanship can be endogenous to each other as some presidents increased their popularity due to strict measures and the framing of their achievements, a phenomenon known as the rally-round-the-flag effect (Klobovs, 2020; Natal, 2021; Sosa-Villagarcia & Hurtado Lozada, 2021; Tagina, 2021).

Calvo & Ventura, 2021; Gramacho et al., 2021; Medeiros et al., 2021; Rennó et al., 2021), and Mexico (Bell-Martin & Díaz Domínguez, 2021), among others. The political agency is definitely influential in some cases, so we may use it as a baseline condition or a control variable in statistical models.

As argued in the previous section, political agency should be distinguished from state capacity but may sneak in during the process of policy elaboration and implementation. In the latter case, we closely examine how and to what extent political agency influenced the course of implementation.

Theoretically speaking, the influence of political agency reflects either weak constraints on executives or state apparatus susceptible to political influence. On the one hand, Latin American states have undergone divergent paths in the institutionalization of the policymaking process during the last decades, having some maintain relatively stronger institutional mechanisms of checks and balances while others modified constitutional rules to concentrate power on the executive (Corrales, 2018; Flores-Macias, 2012; Stein & Tommasi, 2008). This is a discussion of how political choice disturbs the direct translation of state capacity into policy outcomes.

On the other hand, Latin American states are known to be permeable to political maneuvers, leaving vast parts of policy processes in clientelist, corrupt, or biased operation (Calvo & Murillo, 2013; Yashar, 2018), which many states fought to tackle for a long time (Geddes, 1996; Wise, 2003). Auyero (2012) illustrates how unevenness and uncertainty in street-level bureaucrats reproduce exclusive and non-institutionalized states. Contrary to the first type, this is a matter of policy implementation and, hence, a source of state capacity limitations in Latin America.

In this regard, we concentrate on state capacity rather than political agency and claim the merits of the former for the study of the COVID-19 pandemic. Political agencies are certainly decisive in crafting policies in the short run and could also shape the initial step for state-building. Focusing mostly on this short-term element, however, cannot provide meaningful lessons, as our main goal is to know how people can be better prepared in any future circumstances, regardless of leadership at the moment.

1.5.2 Societal Explanations

Another explanation for outcome variations relative to the COVID-19 pandemic looks more toward societal reasons than the states. From the onset of the pandemic, scholars have argued that the compliance and conformity of people toward state-led containment measures were associated with trust in government, risk-averse cultures, uneven social backgrounds, and political beliefs among citizens (Bargain & Aminjonov, 2020; Cairney & Wellstead, 2020; see also literature on political agency). Specifically, Anttiroiko (2021: 12) suggests that better preparedness in East Asia was not only due to the strong states and the recent experience of SARS but also a civil society that "shows high level of conformity and norm compliance, which is an obvious precondition for successful social distancing and lockdowns."

In the Latin American context, pre-existing inequalities and vulnerabilities among the population may provide a reason for the severe outcome. Societal explanations tend to direct attention toward different social realities associated with socioeconomic inequality, informality, and housing and living conditions (Bargain & Aminjonov, 2021; Bottan et al., 2020; Carreras et al., 2021). "Non-salaried, unprotected workers and their families have been disproportionately affected" (Hummel et al., 2021, e580) since they did not afford conditions for remote work, lived in overcrowded spaces, and lacked formal social protections. Extant reports inform how disproportionately people in informal work environments and lower socioeconomic strata were more affected by compulsory confinement measures (Busso et al., 2020; Mancini, 2021).

Nonetheless, not all unequal societies, like Latin American countries, report the same policy measures or outcomes as the chapters in our collection demonstrate. Cross-national variations are rather indicative of long-term trends among our Latin American cases, alerting the importance of structural conditions that evolved over time. Moreover, a weak state capacity is not the end of our analysis. While the highly unequal society, together with low trust in government, suggests low compliance with state measures to contain coronavirus spread, societal reactions should not always be regarded as passive or counterproductive. We turn to this point in the next section.

1.6 Responding to Weak State Capacity

As widely acknowledged, Latin American states are often not strong and rather permeable to political influence, as discussed earlier. So, approaching from the state capacity perspective, we look beyond the evaluation of state strengths and weaknesses. Even if we observe that a national state is weak in implementing policies, it cannot fit into a single conclusion. Burgeoning studies based on the Latin American experience made pivotal breaks in the theoretical understanding of limited implementation capacity and state weaknesses (Amengual, 2016; Brinks et al., 2020; Holland, 2017; Hummel, 2021). We draw two major strands of arguments from the literature for the sake of our discussion on the pandemic: subnational variation and collaborative governance.

The first argument assumes that the state capacity and policy implementation involve interactions by multiple governments. Responses to the pandemic are often a question of multi-level governance involving centralization in decision-making, federalism, and inter-governmental coordination (Béland et al., 2021; Bromfield & McConnell, 2021; Cyr et al., 2021; Schomaker et al., 2021; Steytler, 2021). After the waves of decentralization in the late twentieth century, primary healthcare services have often been in the hands of subnational tiers, although some kinds of national-level decision-making also mattered.

We take a closer look at the subnational variation and national-subnational coordination since the knowledge gap may derive from this point. During the pandemic, cooperation among governments at different levels and municipalities at the same level created uneven policy implementation outcomes (Arias Yurisch et al., 2020; Ramírez De La Cruz et al., 2020). The subnational comparisons in China (Ji et al., 2020) and Brazil (Schaefer et al., 2020) showed significant associations between health service preparedness and health outcomes. In contrast, the same association is not apparently present in cross-national comparisons in the Latin American region (Cameron et al., 2023).

The second argument looks beyond governments and considers the interaction between the state and social actors or among social actors. We depart from fully societal explanations but incorporate uneven patterns of collaboration in the state-society relationship as a vital sphere of the policy implementation process. Although under different terms across scholarly fields, like social innovations (Calò et al., 2024), co-creation (Amengual & Dargent, 2020; Scognamiglio et al., 2023), and co-production (Carminati et al., 2023), many scholars have echoed similar concerns. We align with the suggestion by Cyr et al. (2021) that collaboration between the state and non-state actors is a possible channel through which the states achieve the ideal policy implementation. Undoubtedly, support from epidemiologists and other experts was crucial in designing and implementing policies. The supply of essential materials and their distribution to marginalized people were usually carried out through organizations and actors in civil society. Giraudy et al. (2020) argue that labor unions in Argentina enabled a stricter lockdown, and federalism in Brazil and Mexico produced variegated responses across states.

1.7 Methodological Approaches

Our goal is to provide answers to the three questions that reveal gaps, which need diverse approaches in the methodological sense. Studies on the COVID-19 pandemic have to tackle both epidemiological phenomena and political and social factors that are associated with them. This means that chapters in our book must carefully measure health outcomes and state capacity, multi-faceted and multi-dimensional in each. Also, to assess the explanatory power of state capacity on the state responses and health outcomes, we should deploy comparative analysis across national, subnational, and individual units, as well as inter-temporal variations. This makes analytical eclecticism inevitable to deal with complex social phenomena, as we wish to contribute with enhanced theoretical and analytical rigor (Rezende, 2021).

The state responses to the pandemic range from a variety of issues, some of which are institutional, while others are behavioral. We focus on the primary measures needed to mitigate the health risk, i.e., testing, mask-wearing, lockdown, social distancing, and vaccination. In other words, we set aside secondary policies to reduce collateral damages, such as income losses, economic vulnerabilities, and mental distress caused by the primary measures.[7]

Table 1.2 summarizes the focus of seven analytical chapters and the cases, data, and analytical strategies they adopt. Chapters 2–5 mainly address the first research question, focusing on issues such as health regimes, testing capacity, mask-wearing compliance, and subnational variation in health infrastructures. Chapters 6–8 mostly correspond to the second research question, focusing on policy emulations, collaborative governance (and lack thereof), and vaccine development in state-society collaboration.

To be precise, each chapter not only responds to one of the three questions but also draws some insights for other questions as well. Therefore, we knit together lessons and findings from all chapters to synthesize our answers to all the third research questions in Chap. 9.

The data, cases, and analytical strategies the chapters adopt are also heterogeneous, depending on the issue's nature, data accessibility, and analytical advantages. Some attempt to address the state capacity conceptually based on the behavioral data that illustrates its manifestation. Others examine state capacity in the broader institutional setting, like health regimes of the welfare states at national and subnational levels. Our approach is multi-method, embracing "inferential pluralism" (Rezende, 2021), applying the most desirable analytical strategy as best suited for the research subject in each dimension.

Table 1.2 Focuses and methodological approaches of each chapter

	The analytical focus	Cases, data, analytical strategy
Q1 What do state strengths and weaknesses explain about the responses and outcomes to the COVID-19 pandemic?		
Chap. 2	Divergence in health regimes	Regional comparison, national-level statistics, correlation
Chap. 3	Gap in testing capacity	Regional comparison, daily survey data, correlation and QCA
Chap. 4	Mask-wearing compliance	Regional comparison, daily survey data, regression discontinuity design and QCA
Chap. 5	Path dependency of subnational divergence	Brazilian subnational analysis, state-level statistics, descriptive inference
Q2 What solutions were practically available when state capacity was weak or limited?		
Chap. 6	Policy emulation among regional peers	Regional comparison, presidential decrees, text analysis and regressions
Chap. 7	Weak collaborative governance	Selective case studies, fieldwork, critical analysis
Chap. 8	Vaccine development	Argentina, fieldwork, process tracing

Source: Author
QCA qualitative comparative analysis

[7] This is an ideal-typical distinction since any containment measures are usually balanced with collateral damages and accompanied by compensatory measures. For the studies of secondary politics, see Blofield et al. (2020) and Blofield (2023) for example.

By the same token, we don't set any scope limits territorially or temporarily. The analytical level may differ from national to subnational and individual levels. Some concentrate on a specific country case, while others are cross-national analyses. The time scope can range from the first months to the first year or 2–3 years from the onset, depending on the research rationale of the focused issue, and then trace back to antecedents as much as needed.

While methodological approaches may vary chapter by chapter, we follow a couple of methodological guidelines as common benchmarks. First, as explained in the previous sections, we contest that general state capacity indicators commonly used by the previous works can only give an incomplete answer. While such a quick solution may help to signal what's worth exploring further, a more careful assessment of the actual gap in capacity is warranted. Although some chapters rely on suboptimal indicators, others identify more nuanced alternatives.

Second, all chapters deploy comparative perspectives that propose arguments with a broader implication beyond a single case. This does not necessarily require working in more than one country. State capacity variations can be assessed not only across countries but also within a country, across subnational units, or over time. Still, similar to previous studies using state capacity, filtering long-term capacity from short-term confounders is always a mission for empirical analyses. We ensure that a direct comparison among cases or a careful examination of counterfactual possibilities is carried out to distinguish what belongs to state capacity from what does not. Due to the data accessibility, this book principally draws lessons from some countries where data is more accessible, but the lessons from those countries are expected to travel to other countries in the region and globally.

1.8 The Organization of Chapters

The book is composed of nine chapters. Following this first one, Ilan Bizberg and Mauricio Jiménez Hernández in Chap. 2 introduces the regional landscape of health regime structure and divergence among Latin American countries, which provides a background and overview of the regional context before proceeding to the following chapters. Moreover, a correlational analysis in his chapter points out that health infrastructure, such as the number of doctors and intensive care units per population and disposable health expenditure, explains the mortality related to COVID-19 infection. Simply put, the more institutionally equipped a country was, the less severe the damage it had. While unique political agencies in a few countries like Brazil and Mexico add other nuances to the comparative landscape, he confirms that state capacity is one of the major explanations that illustrate cross-national variations.

In Chap. 3, Isamu Okada problematizes the measurability of state capacity during the COVID-19 pandemic by focusing on the capacity to implement tests. Tests are supposed to flag the primary identification of virus infection, which is a baseline that all other observations should rely on—whether any events that happened are certainly related to COVID-19. Notwithstanding, the test accuracy is subject to capacity limitations, and hence, official data does not always represent the facts. Against this backdrop, this chapter takes advantage of daily survey data collected by the University of Maryland and Meta—the same as Miyachi's Chap. 4. This data directly approaches citizens' self-reported experience, which enables an observation of test capacity limitations that circumvents measurement bias due to the very state capacity. The chapter not only measures the test capacity limitations among Latin American countries but also checks how much the capacity limitation indicator can explain health outcomes, such as case fatality rates.

Chapter 4 gears our attention toward mask-wearing compliance, a typical non-pharmaceutical measure against the COVID-19 infection. Takahiro Miyachi, the author of this chapter, sheds light on the citizens' mass-level behavior as a dependent variable, which is distinctive from other chapters. His mixed-method approach that combines the regression discontinuity design and qualitative comparative analysis illustrates that state announcement is not something that dictates citizens to perfectly follow mask-wearing compliance but a complementary tool that encourages them to wear masks when many people had still not been wearing masks and the infection trends show uncertainty, declining or remaining stable.

Chapter 5, by Shuichiro Masukata, takes another perspective to state capacity variations through a cross-subnational and longitudinal observation. His chapter narrates the evolution of the Unified Health System (*Sistema Único de Saúde,* SUS) in Brazil, one of the most advanced primary health care systems in the region. While this system has been fundamental, subnational disparities were evident and possibly path-dependent. He suggests that the subnational region lagged in the system in terms of infrastructure, expenditure, and basic conditions reported severe impacts during the pandemic.

While these four chapters address empirical manifestations of state capacity variations, the following chapters focus on what happens under weak state capacities. Chapter 6 by Hirokazu Kikuchi provides another lesson related to quick responses at the onset of the pandemic. His perspective is unique and insightful; when a state lacks sufficient capacity to tackle urgent challenges, it may imitate what other regional peers do for the same issue. The chapter uses an original dataset comprised of 159 presidential decrees issued in February–March 2020 in 12 Latin American countries. A combination of text analysis and dyad data regression proves that low health service delivery and administrative capacities matter to the chance of emulation between two regional pairs.

In Chap. 7, Matias Bianchi, Florencia Coda, and Sofia Santamarina map out the cases of collaborative governance societal responses to the pandemic in six countries, namely Argentina, Bolivia, Chile, Colombia, Guatemala, and Mexico. Their interpretation, however, is critical, highlighting obstacles and challenges. During the COVID-19 pandemic, collaborations between the state and society were, by and large, ad hoc and short-lived. Common negative factors, like political instability and low trust in state entities, overshadowed the possibilities of collaborative governance that could have moved to institutionalize societal endeavors.

In Chap. 8, María Cecilia Sanmartín and Gabriela Bortz provide a contrasting picture of successful public–private collaboration in the vaccine development in Argentina. It started with the delayed arrival of the COVAX-supplied vaccine, but then private firms offered the chance of analytical technology transfer to the Argentinean Drug Regulating Agency (ANMAT) about Sputnik V in early 2021, which complemented the delay. This and other earlier reinforcements of state agencies enabled further success. From 2022 to 2023, the state-sponsored initiatives that involved a public university and private firms resulted in the production of a COVID-19 vaccine made in Argentina, which is one of the least expensive options nowadays. In this case, the state was present throughout the course of vaccine development during the pandemic, upgrading its capacity and providing research funding to private actors.

Chapter 9 summarizes the main findings in analytical chapters and synthesizes our answers to the three research questions.

References

Alfano, V., & Ercolano, S. (2022). Stay at home! Governance quality and effectiveness of lockdown. *Social Indicators Research, 159*(1), 101–123. https://doi.org/10.1007/s11205-021-02742-3

Alicea-Planas, J., Trudeau, J. M., & Vásquez Mazariegos, W. F. (2021). COVID-19 risk perceptions and social distancing practice in Latin America. *Hispanic Health Care International, 19*(4), 254–259. https://doi.org/10.1177/1540415320985141

Amengual, M. (2016). *Politicized enforcement in Argentina: Labor and environmental regulation.* Cambridge University Press. https://doi.org/10.1017/CBO9781316476901

Amengual, M., & Dargent, E. (2020). The social determinants of enforcement: Integrating politics with limited state capacity. In D. M. Brinks, S. Levitsky, & M. V. Murillo (Eds.), *The politics of institutional weakness in Latin America* (1st ed., pp. 161–182). Cambridge University Press. https://doi.org/10.1017/9781108776608.007

An, B. Y., & Tang, S.-Y. (2020). Lessons from COVID-19 responses in East Asia: Institutional infrastructure and enduring policy instruments. *The American Review of Public Administration, 50*(6–7), 790–800. https://doi.org/10.1177/0275074020943707

Anttiroiko, A.-V. (2021). Successful government responses to the pandemic: Contextualizing national and urban responses to the COVID-19 outbreak in east and west. *International Journal of E-Planning Research, 10*(2), 1–17. https://doi.org/10.4018/IJEPR.20210401.oa1

Arias Yurisch, K., Retamal Soto, K., & Ramos Fuenzalida, C. (2020). COVID-19: Network effectiveness of intermunicipal self-organized response in Chile. *Transylvanian Review of Administrative Sciences, Special Issue, 2020*, 5–23. https://doi.org/10.24193/tras.SI2020.1

Aruguete, N., Calvo, E., Cantú, F., Ley, S., Scartascini, C., & Ventura, T. (2021). Partisan cues and perceived risks: The effect of partisan social media frames during the COVID-19 crisis in Mexico. *Journal of Elections, Public Opinion and Parties, 31*(Suppl 1), 82–95. https://doi.org/10.1080/17457289.2021.1924740

Auyero, J. (2012). *Patients of the state: The politics of waiting in Argentina*. Duke University Press.

Avritzer, L., & Rennó, L. (2021). The pandemic and the crisis of democracy in Brazil. *Journal of Politics in Latin America, 13*(3), 442–457. https://doi.org/10.1177/1866802X211022362

Aydın-Düzgit, S., Kutlay, M., & Fuat Keyman, E. (2023). State capacity and populist rule in times of uncertainty: COVID-19 response in South Korea, Brazil, and Turkey. *Globalizations*, 1–21. https://doi.org/10.1080/14747731.2023.2256567

Bargain, O., & Aminjonov, U. (2020). Trust and compliance to public health policies in times of COVID-19. *Journal of Public Economics, 192*, 104316. https://doi.org/10.1016/j.jpubeco.2020.104316
Bargain, O., & Aminjonov, U. (2021). Poverty and COVID-19 in Africa and Latin America. *World Development, 142*, 105422. https://doi.org/10.1016/j.worlddev.2021.105422
Batista Pereira, F., & Nunes, F. (2021). Media choice and the polarization of public opinion about Covid-19 in Brazil. *Revista Latinoamericana de Opinión Pública*, 1–19. https://doi.org/10.14201/rlop.23681
Béland, D., Marchildon, G. P., Medrano, A., & Rocco, P. (2021). COVID-19, federalism, and health care financing in Canada, the United States, and Mexico. *Journal of Comparative Policy Analysis: Research and Practice, 23*(2), 143–156. https://doi.org/10.1080/13876988.2020.1848353
Bell-Martin, R. V., & Díaz Domínguez, A. (2021). The unmasked electorate: Co-partisanship, personal experience, and perceptions of COVID-19 risk in Mexico. *Revista Latinoamericana de Opinión Pública, 10*(2), 137–162. https://doi.org/10.14201/rlop.26490
Berwick, E., & Christia, F. (2018). State capacity redux: Integrating classical and experimental contributions to an enduring debate. *Annual Review of Political Science, 21*(1), 71–91. https://doi.org/10.1146/annurev-polisci-072215-012907
Bizberg, I. (2024). *Four worlds of the welfare state in Latin America*. Springer International. https://doi.org/10.1007/978-3-031-44420-3
Blofield, M., Giambruno, C., & Filgueira, F. (2020). *Policy expansion in compressed time: Assessing the speed, breadth and sufficiency of post-COVID-19 social protection measures in 10 Latin American countries* (235). Economic Commission for Latin America and the Caribbean (ECLAC). https://www.cepal.org/en/publications/46016-policy-expansion-compressed-time-assessing-speed-breadth-and-sufficiency-post
Blofield, M., Pribble, J., & Giambruno, C. (2023). *The politics of social protection during times of crisis*. Cambridge University Press. https://doi.org/10.1017/9781009416023
Boruchowicz, C., & Lopez Boo, F. (2022). Better than my neighbor? Testing for overconfidence in COVID-19 preventive behaviors in Latin America. *BMC Public Health, 22*(1), 1009. https://doi.org/10.1186/s12889-022-13311-9
Bosancianu, C. M., Hilbig, H., Humphreys, M., Kc, S., Lieber, N., & Scacco, A. (2020). *Political and Social Correlates of Covid-19 Mortality* [Preprint]. SocArXiv. https://doi.org/10.31235/osf.io/ub3zd
Boswell, J., Corbett, J., Rhodes, R. A. W., & Salomonsen, H. H. (2021). The comparative 'court politics' of Covid-19: Explaining government responses to the pandemic. *Journal of European Public Policy, 28*(8), 1258–1277. https://doi.org/10.1080/13501763.2021.1942159
Bottan, N., Hoffmann, B., & Vera-Cossio, D. A. (2020). *The unequal impact of the coronavirus pandemic: Evidence from seventeen developing countries* (IDB Working Paper IDB-WP-1150). Inter-American Development Bank.
Brinks, D. M., Levitsky, S., & Murillo, M. V. (Eds.). (2020). *The politics of institutional weakness in Latin America*. Cambridge University Press. https://doi.org/10.1017/9781108776608
Bromfield, N., & McConnell, A. (2021). Two routes to precarious success: Australia, New Zealand, COVID-19 and the politics of crisis governance. *International Review of Administrative Sciences, 87*(3), 518–535. https://doi.org/10.1177/0020852320972465
Busso, M., Camacho, J., Messina, J., & Montenegro, G. (2020). *The challenge of protecting informal households during the COVID-19 pandemic: Evidence from Latin America* (IDB Discussion Paper 780). Inter-American Development Bank.
Cairney, P., & Wellstead, A. (2020). COVID-19: Effective policymaking depends on trust in experts, politicians, and the public. *Policy Design and Practice, 4*(1), 1–14. https://doi.org/10.1080/25741292.2020.1837466
Calò, F., Scognamiglio, F., Bellazzecca, E., & Ongaro, E. (2024). Social innovation during turbulent times: A systematic literature review and research agenda. *Public Management Review, 26*(6), 1706–1730. https://doi.org/10.1080/14719037.2023.2219998

Calvo, E., & Murillo, M. V. (2013). When parties meet voters: Assessing political linkages through partisan networks and distributive expectations in Argentina and Chile. *Comparative Political Studies, 46*(7), 851–882. https://doi.org/10.1177/0010414012463882

Calvo, E., & Ventura, T. (2021). Will I get COVID-19? Partisanship, social media frames, and perceptions of health risk in Brazil. *Latin American Politics and Society, 63*(1), 1–26. https://doi.org/10.1017/lap.2020.30

Cameron, M. A., Hurtado, V., Sosa-Villagarcia, P., & Gombata, M. (2023). A tale of two crashes: Pandemic politics in Brazil and Peru. *Latin American Perspectives, 50*(4). https://doi.org/10.1177/0094582X231179931

Capano, G., Howlett, M., Jarvis, D. S. L., Ramesh, M., & Goyal, N. (2020). Mobilizing policy (in) capacity to fight COVID-19: Understanding variations in state responses. *Policy and Society, 39*(3), 285–308. https://doi.org/10.1080/14494035.2020.1787628

Carminati, M., Cavenago, D., & Mariani, L. (2023). Co-production before, during, and after the first COVID-19 lockdown: The case of developmental services for youth with disabilities. *International Review of Administrative Sciences, 89*(3), 864–882. https://doi.org/10.1177/00208523221134484

Carreras, M., Vera, S., & Visconti, G. (2021). A tale of two pandemics: Economic inequality and support for containment measures in Peru. *Journal of Politics in Latin America, 13*(3). https://doi.org/10.1177/1866802X211035393

Centeno, M. A., Kohli, A., & Yashar, D. J. (2017). Unpacking states in the developing world: Capacity, performance, and politics. In M. A. Centeno, A. Kohli, & D. J. Yashar (Eds.), *States in the developing world* (pp. 1–32). Cambridge University Press. https://doi.org/10.1017/CBO9781316665657.002

Cingolani, L. (2013). *The State of State Capacity: A Review of Concepts, Evidence, and Measures* (AFD MGSoG/UNU Merit Working Paper Series on Institutions and Economic Growth 53).

Corrales, J. (2018). *Fixing democracy: Why constitutional change often fails to enhance democracy in Latin America*. Oxford University Press.

Cyr, J., Bianchi, M., González, L., & Perini, A. (2021). Governing a pandemic: Assessing the role of collaboration on Latin American responses to the COVID-19 crisis. *Journal of Politics in Latin America, 13*(3), 290–327. https://doi.org/10.1177/1866802X211049250

Dargent, E., Feldmann, A. E., & Luna, J. P. (2017). Greater state capacity, lesser stateness: Lessons from the Peruvian commodity boom. *Politics & Society, 45*(1), 3–34. https://doi.org/10.1177/0032329216683164

Eaton, K. (2017). *Territory and ideology in Latin America: Policy conflicts between national and subnational governments*. Oxford University Press.

Evans, P. B. (1995). *Embedded autonomy: States and industrial transformation*. Princeton University Press.

Fernandez, M., & Machado, C. (Eds.). (2021). *COVID-19's political challenges in Latin America*. Springer International. https://doi.org/10.1007/978-3-030-77602-2

Flores-Macias, G. (2012). *After neoliberalism? The left and economic reforms in Latin America*. Oxford University Press.

Forster, T., & Heinzel, M. (2021). Reacting, fast and slow: How world leaders shaped government responses to the COVID-19 pandemic. *Journal of European Public Policy, 28*(8), 1299–1320. https://doi.org/10.1080/13501763.2021.1942157

García, G. M., Haboud, M., Howard, R., Manresa, A., & Zurita, J. (2020). Miscommunication in the COVID-19 Era. *Bulletin of Latin American Research, 39*(S1), 39–46. https://doi.org/10.1111/blar.13179

Geddes, B. (1996). *Politician's dilemma: Building state capacity in Latin America*. University of California Press.

Giraudy, A., Niedzwiecki, S., & Pribble, J. E. (2020, April 30). How political science explains countries' reactions to COVID-19. *Americas Quarterly*. https://www.americasquarterly.org/article/how-political-science-explains-countries-reactions-to-covid-19/

Gisselquist, R. M., & Vaccaro, A. (2023). COVID-19 and the state: Exploring a puzzling relationship in the early stages of the pandemic. *Journal of International Development, 35*(5), 800–819. https://doi.org/10.1002/jid.3702

Givens, J. W., & Mistur, E. (2021). The sincerest form of flattery: Nationalist emulation during the COVID-19 pandemic. *Journal of Chinese Political Science, 26*(1), 213–234. https://doi.org/10.1007/s11366-020-09702-7

González-Bustamante, B. (2021). Evolution and early government responses to COVID-19 in South America. *World Development, 137*, 105180. https://doi.org/10.1016/j.worlddev.2020.105180

Gramacho, W., Turgeon, M., Kennedy, J., Stabile, M., & Mundim, P. S. (2021). Political preferences, knowledge, and misinformation about COVID-19: The case of Brazil. *Frontiers in Political Science, 3*, 646430. https://doi.org/10.3389/fpos.2021.646430

Greer, S. L., King, E. J., da Fonseca, E. M., & Peralta-Santos, A. (2020). The comparative politics of COVID-19: The need to understand government responses. *Global Public Health, 15*(9), 1413–1416. https://doi.org/10.1080/17441692.2020.1783340

Hanson, J. K., & Sigman, R. (2021). Leviathan's latent dimensions: Measuring state capacity for comparative political research. *The Journal of Politics, 83*(4), 1495–1510. https://doi.org/10.1086/715066

Helmke, G., & Levitsky, S. (2004). Informal institutions and comparative politics: A research agenda. *Perspectives on Politics, 2*(4), 725–740. JSTOR.

Holland, A. C. (2017). *Forbearance as redistribution: The politics of informal welfare in Latin America*. Cambridge University Press. https://doi.org/10.1017/9781316795613

Hummel, C. (2021). *Why informal workers organize: Contentious politics, enforcement, and the state*. Oxford University Press.

Hummel, C., Knaul, F. M., Touchton, M., Guachalla, V. X. V., Nelson-Nuñez, J., & Boulding, C. (2021). Poverty, precarious work, and the COVID-19 pandemic: Lessons from Bolivia. *The Lancet Global Health, 9*(5), e579–e581. https://doi.org/10.1016/S2214-109X(21)00001-2

Ji, Y., Ma, Z., Peppelenbosch, M. P., & Pan, Q. (2020). Potential association between COVID-19 mortality and health-care resource availability. *The Lancet Global Health, 8*(4), e480. https://doi.org/10.1016/S2214-109X(20)30068-1

Klobovs, L. (2020). El impacto del coronavirus en la figura presidencial argentina. *Revista Latinoamericana de Opinión Pública*, 1–24. https://doi.org/10.14201/rlop.23517

Kohli, A. (2004). *State-directed development: Political power and industrialization in the global periphery*. Cambridge University Press. https://doi.org/10.1017/CBO9780511754371

Kurtz, M. J. (2013). *Latin American state building in comparative perspective: Social foundations of institutional order*. Cambridge University Press.

Kurtz, M. J., & Schrank, A. (2007). Growth and governance: Models, measures, and mechanisms. *The Journal of Politics, 69*(2), 538–554. https://doi.org/10.1111/j.1468-2508.2007.00549.x

Lasco, G. (2020). Medical populism and the COVID-19 pandemic. *Global Public Health, 15*(10), 1417–1429. https://doi.org/10.1080/17441692.2020.1807581

Leão, L. S. (2019). A double-edged sword: The institutional foundations of the Brazilian developmental state, 1930–1985. In A. Ferraro & M. Centeno (Eds.), *State and nation making in Latin America and Spain: The rise and fall of the developmental state* (pp. 157–176). Cambridge University Press.

Lindvall, J., & Teorell, J. (2016, October 7). *State capacity as power: A conceptual framework*. The seminar on the State and Capitalism Since 1800, Harvard University.

Liu, Z., & Geva-May, I. (2021). Comparative public policy analysis of COVID-19 as a naturally occurring experiment. *Journal of Comparative Policy Analysis: Research and Practice, 23*(2), 131–142. https://doi.org/10.1080/13876988.2021.1894074

Love, G. J., & Smith, A. E. (2021). Introduction: Politics, public opinion and the COVID-19 pandemic in Latin America. *Revista Latinoamericana De Opinión Pública, 10*(2), 5–12.

Luna, J. P., & Soifer, H. D. (2017). Capturing sub-national variation in state capacity: A survey-based approach. *American Behavioral Scientist, 61*(8), 887–907. https://doi.org/10.1177/0002764217720964

Mahoney, J. (2003). Long-run development and the legacy of colonialism in Spanish America. *American Journal of Sociology, 109*(1), 50–106. https://doi.org/10.1086/378454
Mahoney, J. (2010). *Colonialism and development: Spanish America in comparative perspective*. Cambridge University Press. https://doi.org/10.1017/CBO9780511750328
Mahoney, J., & Thelen, K. A. (Eds.). (2010). *Explaining institutional change: Ambiguity, agency, and power*. Cambridge University Press.
Mancini, F. (2021). Confinement risks and social inequality in Latin America: Evidence from Argentina. *Current Sociology, 69*(4), 471–491. https://doi.org/10.1177/0011392121990018
Mann, M. (1984). The autonomous power of the state: Its origins, mechanisms and results. *European Journal of Sociology, 25*(2), 185–213. https://doi.org/10.1017/S0003975600004239
Mazzuca, S. (2021). *Latecomer state formation: Political geography and capacity failure in Latin America*. Yale University Press.
Medeiros, A., Bertholini, F., & Pereira, C. (2021). Identity versus fear of death: Political polarization under the COVID-19 pandemic in Brazil. In M. Fernandez & C. Machado (Eds.), *COVID-19's political challenges in Latin America* (pp. 133–145). Springer International. https://doi.org/10.1007/978-3-030-77602-2_10
Migdal, J. S. (1988). *Strong societies and weak states: State-society relations and state capabilities in the Third World*. Princeton University Press.
Moisio, S. (2020). State power and the COVID-19 pandemic: The case of Finland. *Eurasian Geography and Economics, 61*(4–5), 598–605. https://doi.org/10.1080/15387216.2020.1782241
Natal, A. (2021). "For the Sake of All, the Poor First": COVID-19, Mañaneras, and the Popularity of the Mexican President. In M. Fernandez & C. Machado (Eds.), *COVID-19's political challenges in Latin America* (pp. 163–181). Springer International. https://doi.org/10.1007/978-3-030-77602-2_12
Niedzwiecki, S. (2018). *Uneven social policies: The politics of subnational variation in Latin America*. Cambridge University Press.
Pagliaro, S., Sacchi, S., Pacilli, M. G., Brambilla, M., Lionetti, F., Bettache, K., Bianchi, M., Biella, M., Bonnot, V., Boza, M., Butera, F., Ceylan-Batur, S., Chong, K., Chopova, T., Crimston, C. R., Álvarez, B., Cuadrado, I., Ellemers, N., Formanowicz, M., et al. (2021). Trust predicts COVID-19 prescribed and discretionary behavioral intentions in 23 countries. *PLoS One, 16*(3), e0248334. https://doi.org/10.1371/journal.pone.0248334
Ramírez De La Cruz, E. E., Grin, E. J., Sanabria-Pulido, P., Cravacuore, D., & Orellana, A. (2020). The transaction costs of government responses to the COVID-19 emergency in Latin America. *Public Administration Review, 80*(4), 683–695. https://doi.org/10.1111/puar.13259
Rausis, F., & Hoffmeyer-Zlotnik, P. (2021). Contagious policies? Studying national responses to a global pandemic in Europe. *Swiss Political Science Review, 27*(2), 283–296. https://doi.org/10.1111/spsr.12450
Rennó, L., Avritzer, L., & Carvalho, P. D. (2021). Entrenching right-wing populism under Covid-19: Denialism, social mobility, and government evaluation in Brazil. *Revista Brasileira de Ciência Política, 36*, e247120. https://doi.org/10.1590/0103-3352.2021.36.247120
Rezende, F. C. (2021). Methodological transformations in contemporary political science. *Política Hoje, 30*(1), 11–39. https://doi.org/10.51359/1808-8708.2021.249802
Sarracino, F., Greyling, T., O'Connor, K. J., Peroni, C., & Rossouw, S. (2024). Trust predicts compliance with COVID-19 containment policies: Evidence from ten countries using big data. *Economics & Human Biology, 54*, 101412. https://doi.org/10.1016/j.ehb.2024.101412
Saylor, R. (2014). *State building in boom times: Commodities and coalitions in Latin America and Africa*. Oxford University Press.
Schaefer, B. M., Resende, R. C., Epitácio, S. S. F., & Aleixo, M. T. (2020). Government actions against the new coronavirus: Evidence from the Brazilian states. *Revista de Administração Pública, 54*(5), 1429–1445. https://doi.org/10.1590/0034-761220200503x
Schomaker, R. M., Hack, M., & Mandry, A.-K. (2021). The EU's reaction in the first wave of the Covid-19 pandemic between centralisation and decentralisation, formality and informal-

ity. *Journal of European Public Policy, 28*(8), 1278–1298. https://doi.org/10.1080/13501763.2021.1942153

Scognamiglio, F., Sancino, A., Caló, F., Jacklin-Jarvis, C., & Rees, J. (2023). The public sector and co-creation in turbulent times: A systematic literature review on robust governance in the COVID-19 emergency. *Public Administration, 101*(1), 53–70. https://doi.org/10.1111/padm.12875

Sebhatu, A., Wennberg, K., Arora-Jonsson, S., & Lindberg, S. I. (2020). Explaining the homogeneous diffusion of COVID-19 nonpharmaceutical interventions across heterogeneous countries. *Proceedings of the National Academy of Sciences, 117*(35), 21201–21208. https://doi.org/10.1073/pnas.2010625117

Segura-Ubiergo, A. (2007). *The political economy of the welfare state in Latin America: Globalization, democracy, and development*. Cambridge University Press.

Serikbayeva, B., Abdulla, K., & Oskenbayev, Y. (2021). State capacity in responding to COVID-19. *International Journal of Public Administration, 44*(11–12), 920–930. https://doi.org/10.1080/01900692.2020.1850778

Silva, P. (2008). *In the name of reason: Technocrats and politics in Chile*. Penn State University Press.

Soifer, H. (2008). State infrastructural power: Approaches to conceptualization and measurement. *Studies in Comparative International Development, 43*(3–4), 231–251. https://doi.org/10.1007/s12116-008-9028-6

Soifer, H. D. (2015). *State building in Latin America*. Cambridge University Press. http://ezproxy.library.qmul.ac.uk/login?url=10.1017/CBO9781316257289

Soifer, H., & Vom Hau, M. (2008). Unpacking the strength of the state: The utility of state infrastructural power. *Studies in Comparative International Development, 43*(3–4), 219–230. https://doi.org/10.1007/s12116-008-9030-z

Sosa-Villagarcia, P., & Hurtado Lozada, V. (2021). Covid-19 and presidential popularity in Latin America. *Revista Latinoamericana de Opinión Pública*, 1–21. https://doi.org/10.14201/rlop.23664

Stein, E. H., & Tommasi, M. (Eds.). (2008). *Policymaking in Latin America: How politics shapes policies*. Inter-American Development Bank. https://doi.org/10.18235/0012350

Steytler, N. (2021). *Comparative federalism and Covid-19: Combating the pandemic*. Routledge. https://doi.org/10.4324/9781003166771

Tagina, M. L. (2021). Presidential approval during the Covid-19 pandemic in Argentina. In M. Fernandez & C. Machado (Eds.), *COVID-19's political challenges in Latin America* (pp. 121–132). Springer International. https://doi.org/10.1007/978-3-030-77602-2_9

Vaccaro, A. (2023). Measures of state capacity: So similar, yet so different. *Quality & Quantity, 57*(3), 2281–2302. https://doi.org/10.1007/s11135-022-01466-x

Velasco-Guachalla, V. X., Hummel, C., Nelson-Nuñez, J., & Boulding, C. (2021). Legitimacy and policy during crises: Subnational COVID-19 responses in Bolivia. *Perspectives on Politics*, 1–19. https://doi.org/10.1017/S1537592721001183

Weiss, L., & Thurbon, E. (2022). Explaining divergent national responses to Covid-19: An enhanced state capacity framework. *New Political Economy, 27*(4), 697–712. https://doi.org/10.1080/13563467.2021.1994545

Wise, C. (2003). *Reinventing the state: Economic strategy and institutional change in Peru*. University of Michigan Press.

Yan, B., Zhang, X., Wu, L., Zhu, H., & Chen, B. (2020). Why do countries respond differently to COVID-19? A comparative study of Sweden, China, France, and Japan. *The American Review of Public Administration, 50*(6–7), 762–769. https://doi.org/10.1177/0275074020942445

Yashar, D. J. (2018). *Homicidal ecologies: Illicit economies and complicit states in Latin America*. Cambridge University Press.

Chapter 2
State Capacity, Divergence in Health Systems, and Outcomes Among Latin American Countries

Ilan Bizberg and Mauricio Jiménez Hernández

2.1 Introduction

The world underwent a pandemic from 2020 to the end of 2021 that strained all its economies and health systems. It was a tragic and exceptional situation that allows us to compare the performance and resilience of the state and try to understand why some countries weathered the crisis better than others. Although the explanations are multifactorial, this paper will concentrate on two factors related to state capacity: the government's attitude to the crisis and the health system's situation. It will analyze the approach that different governments adopted to deal with the pandemic: some governments denied the severity of the disease (Brazil, Mexico), others reacted late (Ecuador, Bolivia), while others did everything they could to face the crisis from the very start (or even prevent it, as soon as the pandemic hit the European countries), like Chile, Costa Rica, Uruguay, and Argentina. This work will also analyze the conditions of the health systems of each country. However, these are not the only elements that explain the effects of COVID-19 on these countries. It may have also depended on the age of their population, their general health situation, the

This chapter uses liberally paragraphs and data from two previous articles by the author:
Bizberg, I. 2022 "Latin American Health Regimes in the Face of the Pandemic," *Interventions Économiques. Papers in Political Economy,* no. 67.
Bizberg, I., 2021 "Politics and the pandemic," ***Interventions Économiques. Papers in Political Economy,*** Hors Série. Transformations.

I. Bizberg (✉)
El Colegio de México, Mexico City, Mexico
e-mail: ilan@colmex.mx

M. J. Hernández
IDESO – UNIGE, Geneva, Switzerland
e-mail: mauricio.jimenez@etu.unige.ch

I. Okada (ed.), *COVID-19 and State Capacity in Latin America*, Latin American Societies, https://doi.org/10.1007/978-3-032-15572-6_2

country's geography, its links to the world economy—particularly China—the origin of the pandemic, and others.

The health crisis that hit the world in December 2019 and Latin America head-on in March 2020 was a terrible tragedy that claimed millions of lives. Nevertheless, it was also an opportunity to measure the performance of the various governments and health regimes of the continent, a type of social experiment, as it was a unique event that simultaneously affected all the world's countries. As this event puts into question the individual countries' internal situation, it can be used to measure how they reacted to the event from various perspectives. It allows social scientists to analyze how different demographic, health, social, and political situations determine the internal consequences of the pandemic. For this study, I will limit my focus to the two aforementioned causes, governmental attitude and the health system's situation, to discover how they can explain the crisis from the perspective of state capacity.

In this article, I follow the definition of state capacity as stated in the introduction of this book, which is not the "...power by the state elite itself over civil society [but rather] power of the state to penetrate and centrally co-ordinate the activities of civil society through its infrastructure" (Mann, 1984, p. 190). State infrastructures give the state the capacity "to penetrate civil society and to implement logistically political decisions throughout the realm" (Mann, 1984, p. 190). This implies what Soifer, following Mann, calls institutional power rather than infrastructural, which defines "the State's ability to implement its chosen policies" (Soifer, 2015, p. 10); that is, "the ability of the State to induce residents, firms, and organizations to act in ways they would not in the absence of its regulatory and administrative presence" (Kurz, 2013, pos. 129). It is also what Soifer considers as "the ability of the state to exercise control and implement policy choices throughout the territory it claims to govern," stressing the "territorial reach of state institutions, or the ability of the state to consistently and effectively perform a set of core basic functions throughout its realm" (Soifer, 2015, p. 9).

Thus, state capacity is not strength or control but, according to Mann (1984), the aptitude to make decisions and implement them in a particular territory. This capacity requires a certain penetration or embeddedness in civil society. Evans (1995) considers this as the capability of states to pursue a country's development, which requires the state's cooperation with entrepreneurs to develop specific sectors of the economy. It is also called the competence to implement policy choices or induce actions.

Referring to Mann's two definitions of state power is helpful for our purpose. One "is the despotic power of the state elite, the range of actions which the elite is empowered to undertake without routine, institutionalized negotiation with civil society" (Mann, 1984, p. 188). The other is institutionalized power, which is more and more present, substituting despotic power when the second type of power is constructed: "The power of the state, especially in today's capitalist democracies... [is] infrastructural power, the capacity of the state to actually penetrate civil society and to implement logistically political decisions throughout the realm" (Mann, 1984, p. 189).

This definition of state capacity based on its institutions implies that the state is both an arena and an actor. It is an arena, not so much in the sense of one where different sectors of society try to impose themselves to make decisions, but, instead, of a "territory bounded and naturalized," where "the states gradually acquired far greater infrastructural powers: taxation, a monopoly over military mobilization, permanent bureaucratic administration, a monopoly of law-making," (Mann, 1984, p. 209) but also education, health, economic infrastructure, etc.

However, the state is also an actor actively involved in developing a country economically, controlling its population, or defending it during a military, economic, or health-related crisis. The capacity of the state to act within the confines of a territory is based on its infrastructure, its legitimacy, and the ability of its government to use both legitimacy and infrastructure to make decisions that help implement concrete actions. While legitimacy is based on a social compromise, which can be broader or more restricted, allowing the state more or less ability to act, its capacity also depends on the institutions of the state, their solidity and reach, and the government's aptitude to mobilize them.

This chapter agrees with Jassanoff et al. (2021) that, facing the pandemic, the governments that acted most adequately were those that could either impose "top-down" measures without contestation (for example, dictatorial governments such as China or centralized countries such as France) or those that depended on their legitimacy and authority (as defined by Arendt, 1954), such as Germany and New Zealand. In contrast, countries where the social compromise was broken, polarization abided, and the governments either sided with one sector of society against another or did not take the pandemic seriously were the ones that managed the pandemic the worst (United States, Brazil, Mexico, and Peru). While the more authoritarian countries efficiently used their state capacity to manage the crisis and either reinforce their authoritarian power or introduce some authoritarian measures to their regimes, the authoritative regimes, based on a broad consensus, transparency, and authority, used their state competence, not only to manage the crisis successfully but also to reinforce democracy.

The countries where their government defended the "thesis that COVID-19 was the result of some conspiracy, or that the scientific community was wrong, or that the coronavirus was not as serious as it was believed to be, or that masks, quarantines, and vaccines were not necessary, countries such as the United States, England, Brazil, Argentina, [and Mexico that] were left helpless for a time in the face of the pandemic" (Arroyo Laguna, 2023) were the ones who wasted their state capability and failed to stand up to the health crisis.

Based on these definitions of the characteristics of state capacity, this chapter will analyze how several Latin American states managed the health crisis caused by the coronavirus from three different perspectives. On the one hand, as state capability depends on a series of institutions, their solidity, and the ability to coordinate their actions, it is evident that, in the face of a health crisis, the health system is crucial and fundamentally concerned with its population coverage. Coverage here means its extension throughout the territory and its population, as well as its equity and its aptitude to assure all the population of more or less equal treatment when facing health problems. Both aspects diverge in various countries and explain the different abilities of the state to face the health crisis.

On the other hand, as previously mentioned, state capacity also depends on governmental competence and the government's will to use the state's institutions and authority. Governmental competence does not always coincide with state capacity. To understand this fact, one may look at Great Britain, the United States, Mexico, and Brazil, which just "lived through" the pandemic, as opposed to Germany, New Zealand, Uruguay, and Costa Rica.

In this respect, this work will analyze the response of some of the governments in Latin America in assuring the population, transmitting the correct messages in order to protect their population from becoming sick, the attitude of the government, the seriousness with which it took the pandemic, and the right messages it sent to the population. On the other hand, the concrete measures these governments took to sustain families' jobs and financial resources averted people from risking their lives. Too little support for the economy, especially in countries where the informal sector is enormous and the population lives day-to-day, leads to people taking life risks during a pandemic, such as the one we lived through from 2020 to 2022.

We have said that state capacity depends on the breadth and reach of the state's infrastructure and institutions. The health system is the most crucial institution in managing a health crisis. State capability with regard to health can be defined as: (1) Coverage—the reach of the state institutions to the population in terms of the percentage of the population that has access to some health care, be it social security (based on a formal job, contributions, etc.), state-administered services for the general public, or private, insurance or services; (2) state health capability, also defined by the breadth of the system's infrastructure, which is crucial (e.g., how many doctors, nurses, and regular and intensive unit beds); and (3) the system's homogeneity and equity, determining the scope of the state infrastructure.

2.2 The State and the Political System

Most of the governments in the world implemented extraordinary measures during the pandemic. On the one hand, dictatorial/totalitarian systems, such as China, managed to effectively tackle the health crisis at the beginning with extreme measures to restrict the movements of the population. China had been perfecting its population control mechanisms to establish a political system dominated by one party for several years. Turned into a totalitarian system, these mechanisms allow the state to accumulate centralized information about its population, which allows it to exercise control over each individual, not only to recognize political opponents but also to determine acceptable standards of behavior. However, although this model was successful in dealing with the pandemic at the beginning, the situation became economically and socially untenable when the aim of the government changed to controlling the population instead of the pandemic, continuing with its zero-COVID strategy for almost 3 years. Although it seemed to help the government to perfect its control mechanisms, it finally displayed itself as frail, unable to grasp that a health crisis cannot be managed only through control. A certain acceptance from the population to take care and be vaccinated is necessary, as we can see from the example of democratic countries.

Some democratic governments, such as France, Argentina, Uruguay, and Peru, among others, imposed highly restrictive measures on individual liberties during the pandemic. It would have been impossible to take these measures a few weeks earlier. This form of government was fragile during the pandemic, as it was obliged to impose anti-democratic measures, which, as discussed above, may poison the regime from the inside. These measures may serve to reinforce others that had been facing a terrorist risk, which increased since the destruction of the Twin Towers in New York.

Other democratic governments did not impose drastic control measures but based their reaction to the crisis on authority and the population's trust in its government. Not only may this form have been the most effective in managing the crisis and preserving the population's health, but it also managed to avert the imposition of restrictive measures and succeeded in deepening democracy and individual liberties. The governments built their foundations on truthful information, the confidence of the population in its leadership, and the voluntary acceptance of all measures to preserve the population from the virus.

These three modes of dealing with the crisis were achieved in countries with relatively high state capacity. Some countries implemented their institutional power in a dictatorial manner, such as in the case of China, including some degree of authoritarian measures like curfews, prohibition to move away from their domiciles more than a certain distance (France, Italy, Argentina, and Peru), or gather with more than a limited number of people in their homes or outside. Other countries that not only had a high level of the infrastructural state but also a high level of legitimacy and trust in their population, such as Germany, New Zealand, and, partially, Argentina, Uruguay, and Chile, did not impose almost any measures, confident in giving their citizens truthful information upon which they would behave accordingly.

In contrast to these three ways different types of governments reacted to the crisis, populist governments failed to combat the pandemic efficiently, as seen in the United States, Brazil, Great Britain, and Mexico. The Populist-led regimes rest on a reciprocal relationship of faith between the leader and the people that does not rely on institutions. They did not take the health emergency seriously. The United States and Britain had the state infrastructure to respond efficiently. However, their leadership did not act responsibly due to its posture and lack of faith in the institutions that mediate between the population and the government.

In political terms, China can be considered the country that has advanced the most in controlling or administering its population. It has achieved this through the state's capacity to threaten its citizens credibly and use various control instruments such as monitoring mass media, censorship of social networks, access to cell phones and other private press, access to electronic payment data, and facial recognition. The information collected due to the transition from a cash economy into a digital economy allows the government to know what individuals buy, if they pay their debts on time, and if and where they travel. The government can discern each person's interactions by matching individual data with other consumers (something that has been perfected during the pandemic to detect contacts of those infected). Before the current health crisis, the central government used these mechanisms not only to prevent crime, as in democratic countries, but also to identify political opponents. Using these surveillance instruments, the Chinese government began to rank individuals based on their observance of social rules, allocating "social credits" to individuals to give discounts on public transportation, hotels, and other activities to those positively ranked. On the contrary, for those negatively ranked, the government obliged them to pay more for those events or barred them from going to the theater or traveling somewhere on vacation (Han, 2020).

Until the beginning of 2023, the health crisis seemed to confirm this idea and the efficacity of the regime. Nonetheless, this system finally showed its frailties. The control mechanisms continued and were even reinforced without relation to the pandemic. What had worked well initially continued even after the vaccines were invented and expanded in their use in 2022, even though the health crisis was averted. As it was demolishing the second element of the social compromise that the dictatorial state had with its population (economic growth through the continuous lockdowns), this authoritarian system reached its limits. It lost the capacity to be critical of its methods and to convince the population to do what had to be done at some moment of the pandemic.

The measures available to democratic governments assumed the imposition of restrictions that would have been unthinkable a few weeks before the pandemic. Some democratic countries implemented movement limitations that were unimaginable before: they forced citizens to stay home, required them to have a safe-conduct to go to the pharmacy, the corner store, or to exercise, and even defined a limit to the distance they could move away from their homes. In some countries, police could fine or even arrest individuals if they could not justify being outside (Bizberg, 2021). In addition, most measures were defined through decrees that did not pass through Congress and did not result from a consensus between parties and the population.

Like many other European countries, France was unprepared to face the health crisis due to the lack of face masks, ventilators, and hospital beds (Germany had twice as many). There was a delay in imposing the measures to curb infections, as the hospital system managed to resist without deciding who to give access to ventilators, as happened in Italy and Spain. However, rigorous and mandatory confinement was imposed, as well as centralized and dirigiste. A notable speech by President Macron symbolized this rigid attitude, describing the fight against the virus as a "war against an invisible enemy" and calling upon a sacred alliance to face it. In contrast, in Germany, in Merkel's equally notable speech, there were no references to war, nor were the measures imposed compulsorily, but rather the cooperation of the population was requested to apply the guidelines for social distancing, as I will discuss below.

The health crisis revealed a manner of confronting the pandemic that does not aspire for greater population control but is based on democratic authority and values. How this political form tackled the health crisis exposed the basis on which it rests: truth, authority, and a democratic and civic culture of the population. The government's message to its citizens was focused on the sheer necessity of radical measures and the need to be respected individually and collectively. This political form was not only the most democratic but also the most successful in tackling the pandemic. In this respect, some of the most exemplary cases were those of Germany, Taiwan, New Zealand, Finland, Iceland, Norway, Portugal, Uruguay, and the province of Kerala in India; women governed several of them.

In Germany, the severity of the situation was recognized and communicated from the beginning. This stands in contrast to dictatorial and populist governments' attempts to hide or withhold information on the gravity of the pandemic, which eroded the population's confidence and, therefore, the effectiveness of the measures once they were decided.

There is a vicious cycle between the imposition of force and the decline of authority. In the case of countries with authoritarian or populist regimes, the measures were applied through authority, as defined by Hannah Arendt (1954). Arendt describes two fundamental characteristics of authority: in the first place, it is the result of neither force nor conviction, and in the second place, freedom is preserved within authority. This means it is unnecessary to convince the population of the correctness of the actions to be taken. However, they are also accepted because they trust the government and its decisions. In contrast, where there is no authority, everything is questioned, and it is necessary to impose the measures forcefully, while failing to enforce them has dire consequences. Arendt also says that the use of force reduces both authority and freedom.

The counterpart of authority is civic culture, the most essential characteristic of democracy for Tocqueville (1835/1981). He wrote that the habit of living in a democracy is more important than the laws themselves; democracy is essentially a tautology insofar as its possibility depends on the existence of democrats. Laws and their authority can only be imposed on citizens willing to follow them; if they are not, you would need a (non-corrupt) police officer behind every one of them. In the cases analyzed in this chapter, authority and civic culture made it unnecessary to impose sanctions to ensure that individuals respect confinement, social distancing, and the use of masks. These measures were implemented without fines or arrests in Japan, Taiwan, South Korea, and Germany. In Japan, Taiwan, and South Korea, there was no need to stop the economy entirely, contrary to countries like Italy, France, Spain, and Argentina.

The very use of masks is proof of this civic culture, as their use in these countries is widespread, not so much as a way to prevent infection but rather to avoid infecting others when sick. Going out in public without a mask when sick would be perceived as a disinterest of others (Han, 2020). In addition, some of these countries had already lived through SARS and MERS, and they based their strategy on carrying out many tests to identify the contacts of those infected and to ask them to isolate and take care of their families.

Angela Merkel's manner of abording the crisis is a clear example of founding the government's response on transparency, authority, and civic culture. There was no talk of war, as in President Macron's speech, but an individual and collective experience of a health crisis. New Zealand's Prime Minister Jacinda Ardern took a similar stance to Merkel's (Bizberg, 2021). Their speeches revolved around the fact that the government intended to be transparent while asking the population for collaboration to stop the pandemic by considering democratic principles and the civic responsibility of the citizens. The acts of government are not an imposition of instructions on individuals that the central state has decided. Nor are these measures to be implemented through the intensification of the control mechanisms of the government, which is the end of deliberation between the different political powers and levels of government. On the other hand, these speeches also make it clear that the main goal was to save lives, that no other principle prevails, that no utilitarian compromise may predominate, and that the government was not looking for a compromise between the economy and health as populist governments attempted.

Alberto Fernández, the president of Argentina, was clear about this fact when he declared in 2020, "The economy has gone through a lot of bad times, and we have recovered, but we will not recover our dignity if we let our countrymen fall into illness and death" (Fernández, 2020). In addition, the government of Fernandez discussed with union representatives and employers the roadmap that public policy related to the health crisis would follow (Bensusan, in press). The president of Uruguay, Luis Lacalle Pou, assured that he did not implement a mandatory quarantine because "he was not willing to advance toward a police state." He explained that "the Uruguayan has a genetic vocation for freedom…Are we not capable of appealing to personal, individual, and collective care in Uruguay? People confined themselves, but not everyone. Those infected were those who were in contact with their relatives. Then we began to reopen construction, random tests were carried out, and there were no infections; rural schools were opened, and there was no difficulty. In June, all students returned to classes voluntarily because it was not mandatory. There is a citizen pact of responsible freedom that my attitudes benefit me and the common denominator. We have gone quite a bit forward and very little backward," he said (Lacalle Pou, 2020).

President Alvarado of Costa Rica spoke of the challenges facing the population in very similar terms to those of Andern in New Zealand (Bizberg, 2021). He declared that "the fight against COVID-19 is tough, it is not over, and there are still several more months to go on this path. These will be tough months and require much responsibility. As a country, we must learn to live during this period, taking care of ourselves from the coronavirus. We cannot let our guard down or let ourselves down. I know that this is not easy. I know that physical distancing causes fatigue and anguish because we cannot hug loved ones. I know many people are very worried because they need to bring sustenance to their homes. I also know that there is concern for health and life because we all fear that a loved one will become infected or be hospitalized. These concerns are also mine. However, I am absolutely certain that this is a brave country, and once again, we will succeed." (Alvarado, 2020). Finally, President Piñera of Chile also emphasized preparedness, transparency, and information: "We are working on a campaign that will allow all citizens to have the necessary information to adopt the best practices … I fully trust that all

Chileans will be able to face with unity and generosity this serious threat to the health of our citizens, whose protection constitutes the priority and concern of our Government and this President" (Piñera, 2020).

In contrast, populist leaders began questioning the gravity of the pandemic, thereby significantly delaying the adoption of measures to deal with it. The main reason these governments acted belatedly is that, as they are based on a very close relationship between the leader and his followers, they depend very closely on performance, which is measured in economic terms. This is why they hesitated long before being convinced (if they ever were) that there were scientific reasons to shut down the economy to save lives. On the other hand, while economic performance is measured month by month, avoiding deaths is not quantified precisely in the context of a pandemic affecting the whole world and where data are missing. The economic slowdown has evident and immediate harmful effects, while the avoided deaths cannot be accounted for precisely. Populist governments tried to hide the death toll, something which was possible in Brazil, Mexico, and Turkey but not in the United States or Great Britain.

On the other hand, insofar as the leader concentrates power and decisions, occupies the totality of the political scene, and thus depends significantly on public opinion, he is hesitant to stop the economy, as he quickly reaps success but also failure. This also prevents him from speaking clearly and transparently about challenges, problems, and mistakes. Moreover, just as they hesitated long before sacrificing the economy, they tried to open it as soon as possible. This led countries under populist leadership, such as Brazil, Mexico, the United States, and Britain, to have the highest number of infections and deaths (Galindo, 2020).

In the case of Mexico, shortly before the health emergency was declared, President López Obrador declared: "There should be no alarm; it is believed that this virus called coronavirus is not so harmful, so fatal. According to the information available, it is not something terrible or fatal. It is not even equivalent to the flu. Look, the coronavirus thing, that you cannot hug; you have to hug, nothing happens. The protective shield is like the *detente* ... The protective shield is honesty; that is what protects, not allowing corruption" (Badillo, D., 2020).

Finally, the most dramatic case was, without any doubt, that of Brazil, whose President Bolsonaro never stopped opposing the point of view of doctors, promoting the idea that confinement was a mistake, making statements contrary to those of his health ministers, and even promoting demonstrations against the confinement measures of his government. He also fired three of his health secretaries for not accepting his ideas and finally appointed a general with no experience in the field as interim minister. He further participated in a manifestation against confinement, saying, "The destruction of jobs by some governors is irresponsible and unacceptable. We will pay dearly for it in the future." (AFP, 2020).

According to the periodical El Pais, "the head of state has repeatedly ignored the recommendations of the Ministry of Health by repeatedly going out into the street, creating crowds, greeting his admirers and taking selfies with them. The mayor of Manaus, the capital of the state of Amazonas, where hospitals are on the verge of collapse, has even accused him of being the main ally of the virus and campaigning against social isolation" (Galarraga Gortázar, 2020).

The executives' attitude toward the pandemic in different countries in Latin America affected the measures taken, especially in the cases of Brazil and Mexico, where populist governments did not take the pandemic seriously and, thus, did not mobilize state capacity to confront its consequences. Unlike most countries, Mexico did not adopt policies to protect formal workers and their enterprises from the effects of the closedowns. Notably, Mexico only included two of the measures signaled by the CEPAL in its 2021 report about the prohibition of dismissal within a short period and regulation of remote work. Compared to other countries, it protected formal and informal employment in the region the least (ECLAC, 2021, as cited by Bensusán, in press). In addition, Mexico is the country on the continent that spent the least—less than 1% of GDP—as displayed in Fig. 2.1 (FMI, as cited in Bensusán, in press).

Although, in terms of measures to support labor, Mexico implemented the prohibition to dismiss workers (as did Argentina, Brazil, Bolivia, and Colombia), it did not implement remote work measures, modifications of the working hours, or use of vacations and temporary suspension of labor contracts, nor did it create licenses for vulnerable workers that most other countries implemented (except Bolivia and Ecuador). Regarding the measures to support the productive structure, Mexico, Bolivia, and Ecuador did not give production stimulus programs or mechanisms to reduce or facilitate the payment of social contributions for employers, nor did they support payroll payments. Finally, concerning policies for social protection for households, Mexico did not implement a program of emergency income, bonuses, and transfers to compensate for job losses. Ecuador and Bolivia did little to support

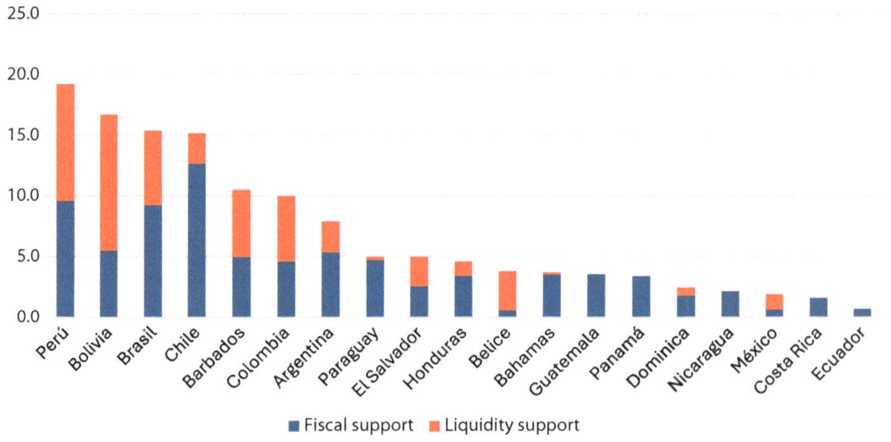

Fig. 2.1 Fiscal support measures as % of GDP in response to the COVID-19 pandemic in Latin American countries. Source: https://www.imf.org/-/media/Files/Topics/COVID/FM-Database/april-2021-fiscal-measures-response-database-publication-mar30.ashx

households, in contrast to most of the continent's other countries (CEPAL, 2021, p. 220–224).

For its part, although Brazil also had a populist leadership, most of the decisions concerning the measures aimed at alleviating the effects of the pandemic were due to multiparty agreements in the National Congress of Brazil, which resulted in implementing the most comprehensive public policy in the region (Bensusán, in press). On the other hand, Brazil's health system is very decentralized due to how the *Sistema Único de Saúde* is organized (Gragnolati et al., 2013). Thus, most of the decisions on restrictions during the pandemic and vaccination were taken at the state level, which mitigated the president's attitude. However, it did not compensate for the deleterious attitude of the Head of State, Bolsonaro, which implied that Brazil did much worse than its health state capability would have prefigured.

In contrast, the countries that reacted seriously to the crisis and mobilized state capacity, such as Argentina, Colombia, and Chile, implemented the most actions to address the socioeconomic effects of the pandemic. They imposed the most restrictions on mobility over an extended period (Bensusan, in press) and spent considerable financial resources. However, while Colombia did much better than expected, Argentina did worse for reasons related to the structure of its health system, as I will discuss in the second part of this paper. In the case of Chile, one of the countries that spent the most to support its citizens and enterprises from the effects of the measures taken to counteract the pandemic, the government implemented significant socioeconomic measures during the first weeks of the pandemic to "…preserve the labor market … protection of jobs and labor income, guaranteeing liquidity for companies, and supporting family income" (Bensusán, in press). Perú also spent a significant number of resources and did much worse. It was facing a political crisis that saw the change of presidencies, and its health system had structural defects, such as a significant number of its citizens without health coverage, much like the other familiarist social protection systems of Ecuador and Bolivia, which I discuss in this paper.

Finally, although Uruguay and Costa Rica spent little compared to other countries, they took the pandemic seriously and had the most solid health capability on the continent. As we can see from Fig. 2.1, they also spent considerable resources supporting households.

Although it is not conclusive, the fact that the attitude based on government authority in many countries—including some Latin American countries—generated a context of trust in the measures announced by the government rendered stricter methods used by more centralized and dictatorial regimes, such as China, useless. On the other hand, countries governed by populist governments ignored the gravity of the pandemic and thus took fewer measures to confront the pandemic. They did not have the support of the population because they ignored the gravity of the situation; the effect of the health crisis was much more profound. We can refer to the data in the introduction to partially confirm this. Meanwhile, countries that implemented populist policies, such as the United States, the United Kingdom, Brazil, and Mexico, had 386, 294, and 378 deaths per 100,000 people, respectively.

Germany, Japan, South Korea, and Uruguay had 251, 114, 120, and 223, respectively, until the end of December 2022 (Our World Data, 2024).

2.3 The Health Systems in the Face of the Pandemic

As mentioned above, institutions are the basis of this book's definition of state capacity. Studying health systems can show how state capability led to better performance during the COVID-19 pandemic. Regarding the health system, I have considered three indicators of state capacity: its coverage, the extent of infrastructure, and its past performance before the pandemic.

In a previous article (Bizberg, 2022), I analyzed how the different structures of the health systems of ten Latin American countries determined the pandemic's consequences in terms of the deaths of their citizens. Using some of the data from my previous article and other information, this chapter analyzes how state capability, as defined in the introduction to this chapter and this book, affected the performance of a set of countries in Latin America during the pandemic.

A health system, one of the principal social infrastructures of the state, along with education, may be robust in terms of its access or coverage, infrastructure, performance, and equity. Different types of health systems may be equally performative. The main exception is what I have called the familiarist health systems, where coverage is low; many families—especially families living in poverty—do not have access to health services, only private ones, and must therefore sacrifice their meager resources on private doctors and medicines. There are three other systems: the statist system, where the state is the central collector of contributions and administers and allocates the services in its clinics and hospitals, and the British NHS and the Latin American, Costa Rican, and Brazilian systems. Socio-corporatist systems are where health is administered and allocated in institutions held by trade unions or mutualist organizations, such as the Argentinian and Uruguayan systems. Finally, examples of systems where private insurance companies and health agencies allocate services are the Netherlands in Europe and Chile and Colombia in Latin America. In the last two types of health regimes, the state has to regulate and equalize the services and allocate them to those incapable of paying for insurance or services. In Colombia, as in the Netherlands, the state subsidizes those who cannot afford health insurance costs and use its services (Schneider et al., 2017; Tikkanen et al., 2020; Bizberg, 2024).

Health systems may be deficient if the difference between the private and public infrastructure and performance is significant. This often happens in Latin America, especially in the commodified health regimes such as the one in Chile or even in the Statist system of Brazil, where private health has been gaining importance. On the other hand, health services may be concentrated in some cities or regions of a country and may be efficient and performative if considered on average but may be very deficient in the countryside or some regions of the country.

With regard to the first indicator, coverage, which is how inclusive the health system is, we can see that the four so-called pioneer countries, as defined by Mesa-Lago (1994), which had achieved a significant expansion before the Second World War (Argentina, Uruguay, Chile, and Brazil), are those which cover almost the entire population. However, two other countries, Costa Rica and Colombia, have recently achieved almost universal coverage: Costa Rica between the end of the Second World War and Colombia with the reforms of the social security system of the Constitution of 1991.

The so-called pioneer countries that developed before the Second World War and reached the majority of the population (around 70%) in the 1970s continue to have higher health coverage, as can be seen in Fig. 2.2, even though their systems have followed different trajectories and coverage is gained by different combinations of the state, social organizations, and the private sector. Nevertheless, there are significant differences regarding the structure of each system, as I began analyzing above, and can be seen graphically in Fig. 2.2. Argentina and Uruguay have preserved a regime dominated by social organizations (unions and mutualists) while developing a state subsystem to cover those not included in a contributive scheme. Only one country, Costa Rica, has succeeded in approaching the pioneer countries with a single, state-run, centralized health model. With the 1988 Constitution, Brazil moved away from its corporatist/segmented trajectory and, like Costa Rica, founded a public structure (the SUS) destined to become the Brazilian NHS, but which, over the years, has left more and more room for the private sector. Finally, even if the military dictatorship in Chile imposed a health scheme dominated by the private

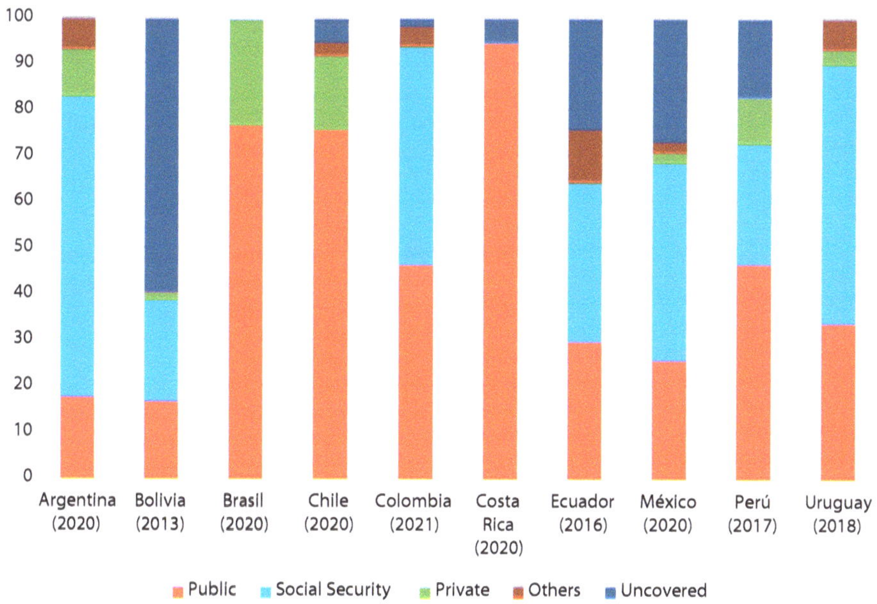

Fig. 2.2 Health system structures. Source: See Appendix

sector, since the democratic transition, it has developed its public service and subjected private health to increasingly strict regulation.

In Table 2.1, I have assessed the situation of the different countries regarding health infrastructure and past performance, with indexes explained in the Annex. Regarding infrastructure, Argentina, Uruguay, and Brazil were the best endowed, Chile, Costa Rica, Mexico, and Colombia were lower, and Ecuador, Peru, and Bolivia were much behind. Regarding past performance, Uruguay and Costa Rica were the best, and then came two other high-infrastructure countries, Brazil and Argentina. Mexico, Chile, and Costa Rica significantly contrast high past performance with relatively low infrastructure. Again, Peru, Ecuador, and Bolivia had the worst past performances.

In general terms, the pandemic has been a humanitarian disaster of significant proportions (Appendix). However, this article has classified the countries of analysis into three groups: Peru, Ecuador, Bolivia, and Mexico, which had (by October 2021) more than 400 deaths[1] per 100,000 inhabitants; an intermediate group formed by Brazil, Argentina, Colombia, and Chile, with deaths between 200 and 355; and the last group of two countries with the lowest rates, Costa Rica and Uruguay, which had less than 200 deaths per 100,000 inhabitants (Fig. 2.3).

The correlation between infrastructure, performance, and number of deaths is very significant. We can see that Uruguay, a country that stands out in infrastructure and performance, also had the fewest deaths during the pandemic. The case of Costa Rica is different, as it has a very high past performance with lower infrastructure. It

Table 2.1 Infrastructure, performance, and excess deaths

(a) Data

	Infrastructure Index	Performance Index	Excess deaths by 100,000 inhabitants
ARG	72.59	79.4	254
BOL	22.87	44.49	416
BRA	58	76.34	355
CHI	42.42	87.65	231
COL	39.93	74.73	326
COS	42.13	84.54	129
ECU	33.33	67.21	435
MEX	39.39	78.19	479
PER	31.38	70.08	707
URU	67.98	85.25	174

(b) Correlations

Infrastructure Index × Performance Index	0.624
Infrastructure Index × Excess Deaths	−0.552
Performance Index × Excess Deaths	−0.516

Source: See Appendix

[1] I will base my evaluation on what has been considered as the most reliable indicator of performance by the health systems: the number of deaths in excess from the last year.

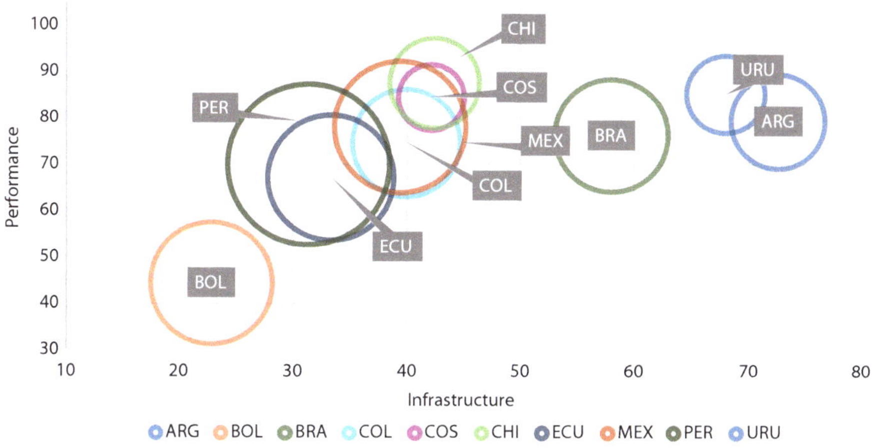

Fig. 2.3 Excess deaths (size of the circles) according to infrastructure and performance. Source: See Appendix

also performed well during the pandemic because its health system is less unequal. Costa Rica has a single-state system and, thus, a more homogeneous system, which, as I will describe below, was a crucial element during the pandemic. Conversely, the countries with the least infrastructure and the lowest performance have had the most deaths: Bolivia, Ecuador, and Peru.

The poor functioning of Mexico's health system during the pandemic, notwithstanding its high past performance, was probably due to deficiencies in infrastructure and the attitude of its government facing the pandemic, which I discussed in the previous section. Although it has a system with a significant social security and public health subsector, out-of-pocket expenditures are the highest in the sample (around 40% of total health expenditure, see Fig. 2.4). This is explained by the fact that a considerable part of the population is without coverage and that total health expenditure is low. We can see in Table 2.2 that both out-of-pocket and total health expenditures are closely related to excess deaths.

The fact that families depend on their means entails that they are pretty helpless in facing health problems and, more understandably, a pandemic like the one we underwent. The fact that health depends so heavily on out-of-pocket expenses means that people hesitate before going to the doctor or the hospital and do so only when their condition worsens; many of the sick approached the clinics when they were seriously ill or died at home.

While the extreme cases can be quite clearly explained, the situation of Argentina, Chile, Brazil, and Colombia require further analysis. The answer to why these systems did not fare as well as one would have expected, according to the indexes of health state capacity while infrastructure and past performance are similar to those countries that fared better, has to do with recent trends in terms of public investment in health (especially in Argentina and Brazil, where the previous governments imposed austerity measures on governmental spending), but especially with the

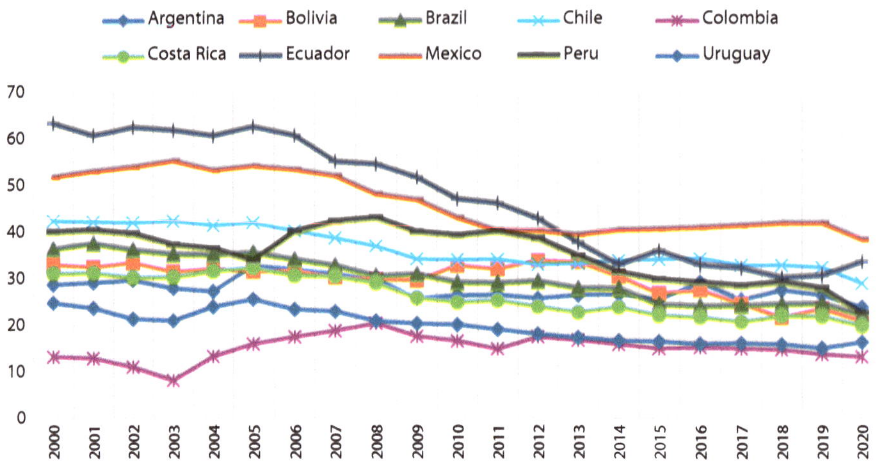

Fig. 2.4 Out-of-pocket health expenditure (% of total). Source: See Appendix

Table 2.2 Correlations with excess mortality

Variable	Correlation with Excess deaths per 100,000 inhabitants
Number of beds per thousand inhabitants	−0.31
Average number of intensive care beds per hundred thousand inhabitants	−0.42
Number of doctors per thousand inhabitants	−0.71
Number of nurses per thousand inhabitants	−0.14
Ventilators per hundred thousand inhabitants	−0.29
Total expenditure on health per capita, PPP	−0.69
Total expenditure on health as a % of GDP	−0.71
Private expenditure on health as % of total health expenditure	0.28
Government expenditure on health as % of total health expenditure	−0.27
Government expenditure on health as % of gross domestic product (GDP).	−0.77
Out-of-pocket expenditure 2017	0.44
GDP growth 2020	−0.80
Percentage of GDP spent on trying to mitigate the economic effect of the pandemic	0.47

Source: See Appendix at the end of the article

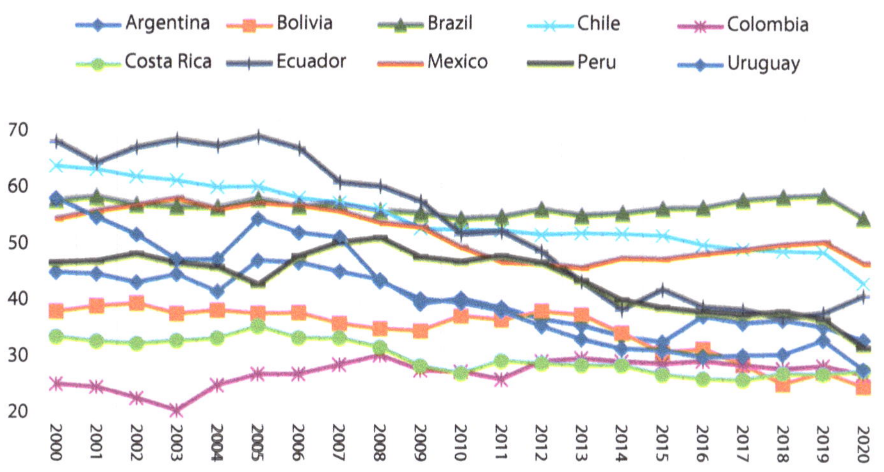

Fig. 2.5 Private health expenditure (% of total health expenditure). Source: See Appendix

structure of the systems: their unequal structure (all of them), and the amount of out-of-pocket expenditure (especially in the case of Brazil and Chile).

While Uruguay and Argentina are very similar in infrastructure and performance, health expenditure as a percentage of GDP, and number of doctors, Argentina did not perform as well as Uruguay in the face of the pandemic. First, during the Macri government (December 2015–December 2019), the social and public health systems deteriorated due to reduced public investment. This fact forced an increase in private health expenditure from a historical low in 2015 (35%) to around 40% in 2018 (See Fig. 2.5). We can see in Table 2.2 that there is a robust negative correlation between the level of total expenditure on health (−0.71) and the government expenditure (−0.77) and a positive one between the proportion of private health expenditure (.28).

Another part of the explanation is the structure of the Argentinian health system. The system is highly segmented, based on the *Obras Sociales* on the one hand and a public subsystem on the other. This segmentation is the source of funding and service quality inequalities, first among the various *Obras Sociales* managed by the unions and then between the public and private systems. Some *Obras Sociales* fare better than others and are generally superior to public services.

On the other hand, there are important regional differences between the capital and the suburbs of Buenos Aires (the *conurbado*) and between the capital and the provinces (Palacios et al., 2020). Financial and infrastructure resources are highly concentrated in Buenos Aires, Cordoba, and Rosario. For example, there are 10.2 doctors and 7.3 beds per 1000 inhabitants in the capital, while in the province of Misiones, there are 1.2 and 1.1, respectively. This explains why the capital had a much better performance (around 30% fewer deaths) than the *conurbado*; while number of beds are not as strongly correlated with the prevention of deaths (−0.31 for regular beds, −0.42 for intensive care beds), number of doctors is highly correlated (−0.71). Another study that also signals geographic inequality centered on cervical cancer and considered it "… a disease symbolic of health inequality; primarily a cancer of the poor, socially vulnerable women, even though there are simple and relatively low-cost means of preventing it" (Arrossi et al., 2008, p. 50). This study found a geographical bias in addition to the rich/educated/labor active/bias, as the mortality rate in the province of Jujuy is almost four times higher than that of Buenos Aires (Arrossi et al., 2008, p. 50). "Women from the Northwestern and Northeastern regions (the least developed areas of the country) were almost three times more likely to be underusers of pap screening […] have the country's highest cervical cancer mortality." (Arrossi et al., 2008, p. 56).

Brazil, with a comparatively well-equipped and performative health system (Table 2.1), also displayed poor performance in the face of the health crisis. On the one hand, there is a significant shortage of doctors akin to that of the familiarist health systems (Fig. 2.6), even if other infrastructure factors are high. This may be part of the explanation, given the strong correlation between number of doctors and deaths. A complementary elucidation is the low level of public expenditure and, therefore, a large proportion of private expenditure, with a significant amount paid out-of-pocket. Brazil is among the countries with the highest level of infrastructure and performance, and yet the one with the most private health expenditure: around 27% (Fig. 2.5).

In addition, like Argentina, there are significant differences in health access between the rural and urban areas and between poorer regions in Brazil (North and Northeast). These characteristics reinforce each other (Figueiredo, 2018). Some

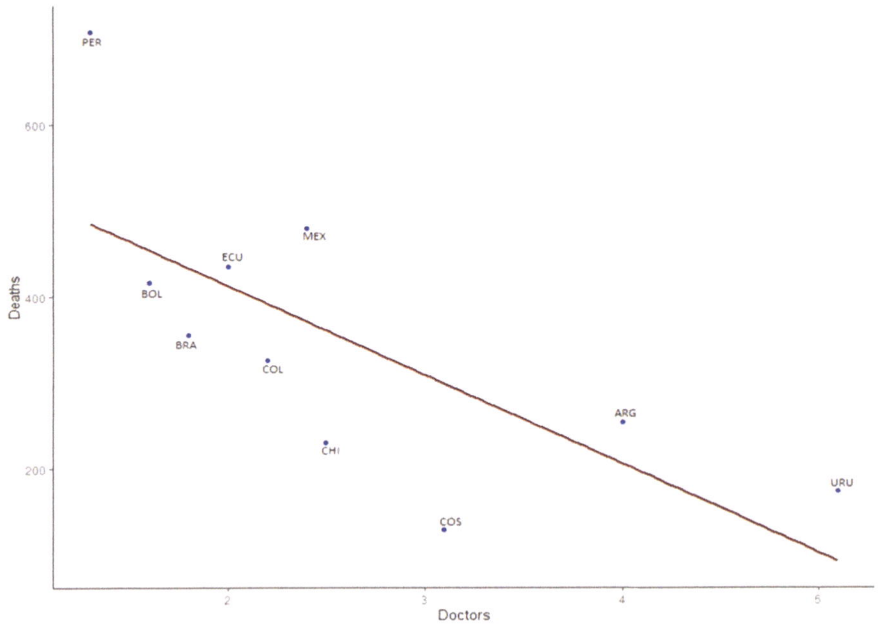

Fig. 2.6 Number of doctors per 1000 inhabitants vs. excess deaths. Source: See Appendix

studies cite one of the primary sources of inequality as the divide between privately insured (25% of the population) and those who rely only on the SUS (Barbosa & Cookson, 2019; García-Subirats et al., 2014). In Argentina, the less effective management of the crisis—compared with Uruguay and Costa Rica—was probably partly due to the segmentation of the health system. However, since Uruguay is also a segmented health system, the additional explanation could be the rural/urban and regional inequalities that coincide with income levels. In Brazil, private insurance has sapped the SUS in addition to these same rural/urban and regional differences (Barbosa & Cookson, 2019).

However, as analyzed in the previous section, another crucial factor to explain the ruinous management of the health crisis is the total irresponsibility of the federal government headed by President Bolsonaro, who never took the health crisis seriously, fought against the confinement, use of masks and vaccines, and made coordination at the national level inoperative (in a manner that is comparable to that which occurred in the United States under Trump). Nonetheless, the governments of some states, such as Sao Paulo and Rio, have managed to cope better. While a federal structure that operates effectively (Canada and Germany) has worked better than many centralized countries (England and France), federal states in which there is no coordination between the federation and the federal states have shown an inferior performance (the United States and Brazil).

Chile is another case that deserves to be discussed at greater length. It is a system that has been reformed by social democratic governments over the past 20 years and has achieved universal coverage. It has a health infrastructure at the top of the performance index. It also has one of the highest total expenditures to GDP (Fig. 2.7). The reasons why Chile failed to measure up to the benchmark countries during the pandemic are similar to those identified in the case of Brazil. Although Chile is a centralized country that does not have Brazil's regional inequalities, it has a similarly high level of private and, especially, out-of-pocket spending (Figs. 2.8 and 2.9). These variables have a robust correlation with deaths during the pandemic. Despite their differences, the Chilean health regime is lopsided toward the wealthy, like all health regimes in Latin America. In the Chilean system, there is a difference between those who have private insurance (and thus also spend more out-of-pocket in a privatized health system such as the Chilean, where insurance fees and co-payments are very high) and those who depend on public health services (Nuñez & Chi, 2013; Vasquez et al., 2013). In fact, according to Vasquez et al. (2013), 79% of the total population is covered by the public health system FONASA, which includes a significant share of the population age 65 or older (87.5%).

On the other hand, 45% of the private ISAPRES beneficiaries, who account for 13% of the total population, belong to the top income quintile. This data shows that FONASA, meaning the government, subsidizes the private sector. On the one hand, ISAPRES concentrates on young, healthy, and wealthy individuals in their productive years, while the public sector concentrates on the old and poor.

Finally, Colombia is also an "outlier" but in a different direction than the three countries I have discussed. It did not fare as badly as expected, considering that it has one of the continent's lowest infrastructure and performance levels and

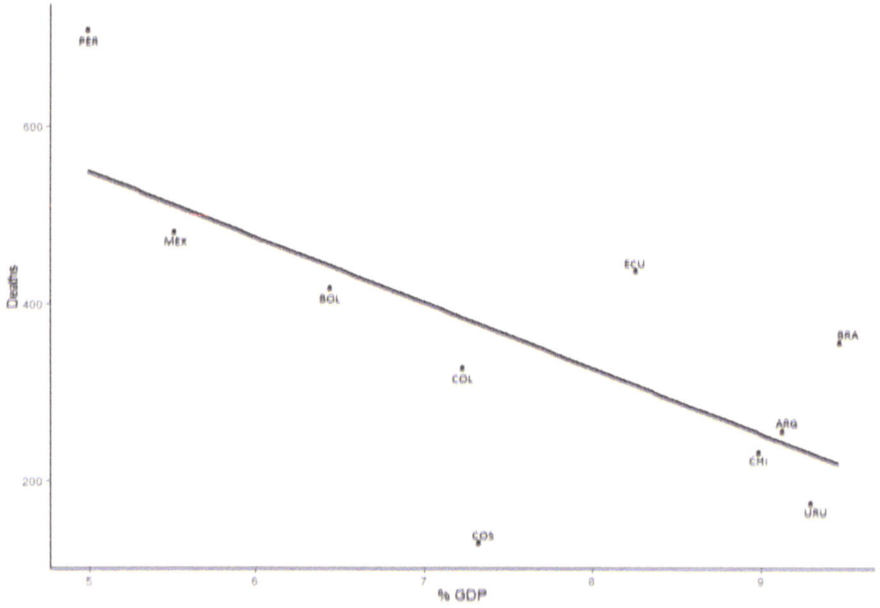

Fig. 2.7 Total health expenditure (% GDP) vs. excess deaths. Source: See Appendix

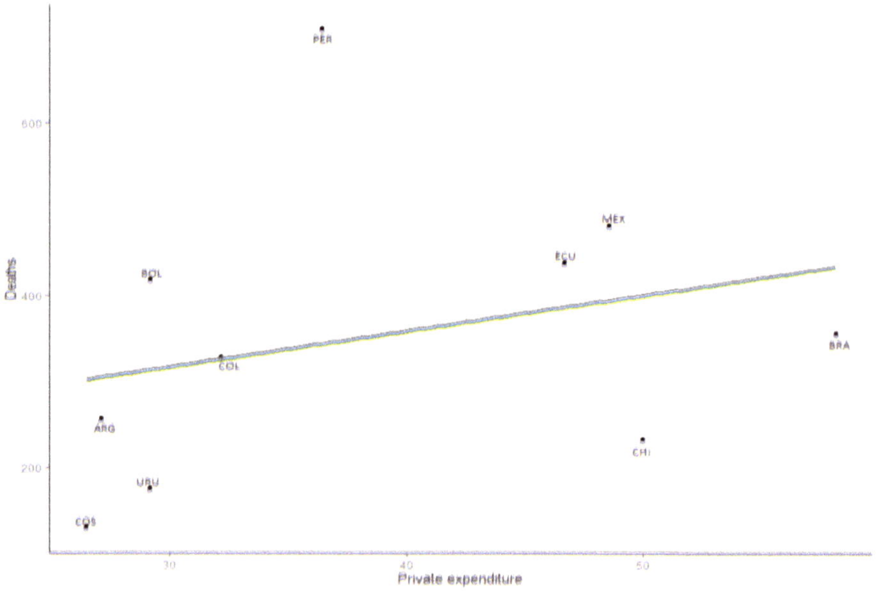

Fig. 2.8 Private current expenditure (% total health expenditure) vs. excess deaths. Source: See Appendix

relatively low total health expenditure (similar to Ecuador, Bolivia, and Peru). It also did not have the number of deaths in these countries or even Mexico (Fig. 2.3). This may be explained by the fact that its health system has succeeded in covering practically its entire population, something that has translated into a very low level of private and (especially) out-of-pocket spending (Figs. 2.4, 2.5, 2.8, and 2.9) both are crucial variables for defining excess deaths. From the discussion on Mexico, Chile, and Bizberg, I., 2021 "Politics and the pandemic," Interventions Économiques. Papers in Political Economy, Hors Série. Transformations, we have learned about the effects of inequality that dependence on private health services and out-of-pocket fees entail.

The Colombian health system can be considered a single-payer system, as the state obliges the population to enroll in either a private or public health plan, concentrates the contributions of all workers, and subsidizes the individuals who lack sufficient resources to pay for their plan. Although it is segmented between a contributive social security system and a subsidized public system—offering different benefits and treating patients in both public and private health centers—and, like the rest of Latin America, has an income bias, it performed better during the pandemic than similar countries in terms of infrastructure and past performance. This was due to reduced private health expenditure and, more importantly (with a higher correlation index), low out-of-pocket expenditure. A study shows that the 1993 reform in Colombia increased the use of preventive and curative outpatient services, a 22% increase in the supply of drugs, and, even more importantly, a 53% reduction in out-of-pocket expenses for outpatients and 50% for inpatients (Ruiz Gómez et al., 2013).

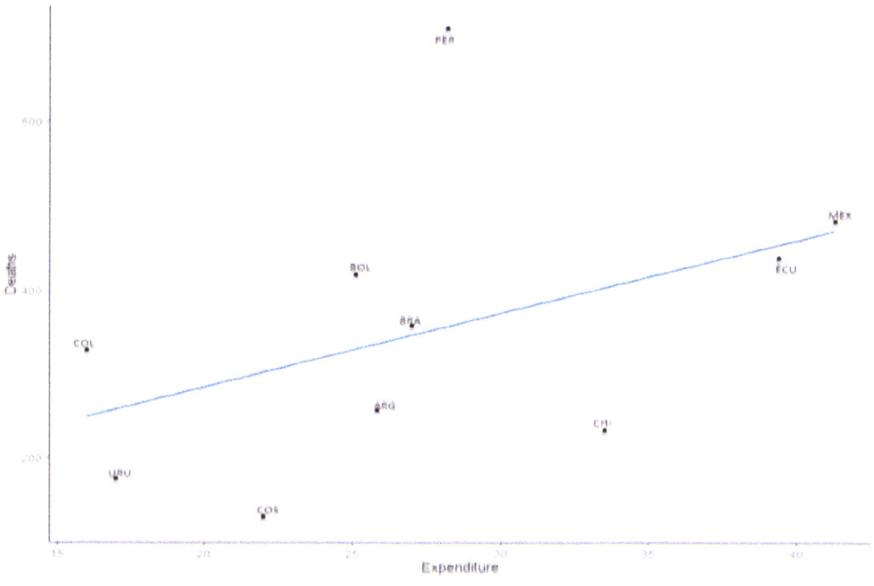

Fig. 2.9 Out-of-pocket expenditure vs. excess deaths. Source: See Appendix

2.4 Conclusions

In order to define the performance of the countries of the Latin American continent in dealing with the COVID-19 pandemic, state capacity, the attitude toward the health crisis, as well as the structure of the health system in terms of coverage, infrastructure, past performance, and equity were all vital to preventing infections and deaths. State capacity was applied through authoritarian or authoritative procedures, either by imposing different restrictive measures or convincing the population to care for themselves. Nonconclusive indicators point to the effectiveness of authoritative rather than authoritarian procedures. Nevertheless, it is clear that those countries that reacted earlier succeeded in implementing tests, mask compliance, confinements, and assistance programs, and providing aid to enterprises in order to keep people at home to mitigate the spread of the virus, as is discussed in the other chapters of this book, most notably Miyachi, Okada, Sanmartín, and Bortz. On the other hand, the countries that had the most solid health institutions suffered less from the health crisis.

Most Latin American governments analyzed in this chapter took the pandemic seriously and tried to implement preventive measures immediately. They did not call for strict confinement because the informal sector on the continent is so large that these measures would have been impossible to implement. When they called for some restriction measures, they economically supported workers and enterprises to keep citizens in their homes. They also advised the use of masks and implemented a broad vaccination.

However, the cases of Mexico and Brazil were an exception. The Mexican president did not take the health crisis seriously at the beginning. Even when the situation worsened and the government began to advise social distancing, it hesitated to conduct tests, impose containment, or advise the use of face masks; in fact, the Mexican president rarely showed himself in public wearing a mask (Sánchez-Talanquer et al., 2020). The case of Brazilian President Bolsonaro is more radical, as he not only avoided advising on mask-wearing and social distancing but also sabotaged these measures when taken by state governments, hindered the purchase of vaccines, and boycotted vaccination. The fact that the governments of AMLO and Bolsonaro did not take the pandemic seriously affected its health system's capacity to deal with the health crisis, which soon overloaded the hospitals and could not cope adequately with the sick.

Concerning the health system's capacity, the most significant indicators that prevented deaths were the number of doctors per capita and the percentage of total health expenditure to GDP; this explains why Costa Rica and Uruguay had the fewest deaths per capita. Countries with the fewest doctors and lowest public spending, like Peru, Bolivia, Ecuador, and Mexico, had many deaths per capita. Other indicators also positively correlate with deaths, such as the level of private and out-of-pocket expenditures. The latter explains why countries such as Brazil and Chile did not fare as well as one could have supposed, according to their relatively high state capacity, as shown by their elevated coverage, strong infrastructure, and high past performance. Despite a relatively high historical performance, Mexico had one of the worst performances in the face of COVID-19. In this case, what played a decisive role was the lack of infrastructure and the lack of coverage (around 30% are not covered), which resulted in a very high out-of-pocket expense (the highest of all the countries considered), in addition to the government's attitude. The contrast with Colombia, which has one of the poorest infrastructures and the lowest performances in the continent, is interesting: Colombia fared much better than Mexico, as almost all of its population is covered by its health system.

Another important element that has affected the performance of health systems is equity. State capacity in the health system structure is measured by coverage, infrastructure level, and performance, but equity is central. The countries that did best facing the pandemic were Uruguay and Costa Rica, both with the least unequal health systems. Despite having one of the best infrastructures, historical performance, and lower out-of-pocket expenses, Argentina performed worse than Uruguay and Costa Rica. This can be explained, on the one hand, by the reduction of investment in health since the commodities crisis, but above all, by the inequities of a highly segmented system that concentrates resources and infrastructure in the capital and some other big cities.

Based on an analysis of the actions of different countries in the face of the health crisis generated by COVID-19, we can conclude that performance at a critical conjuncture depends on state capacity, both in its capacity to implement its decisions through authoritarian or authoritative measures to impose its decisions on society and in the extension and equity of its infrastructure, which are both within Michael Mann's classic definition of state capacity.

Appendix

Sources for Fig. 2.2

ARG: https://www.estadisticaciudad.gob.ar/si/genero/principal-indicador?indicador=tip_cob_sal

BOL: http://www.scielo.org.bo/scielo.php?pid=S1012-29662019000200021&script=sci_arttext

BRA: https://www.commonwealthfund.org/international-health-policy-center/countries/brazil

CHI: https://www.trade.gov/knowledge-product/chile-healthcare

COL: https://www.minsalud.gov.co/proteccionsocial/Paginas/cifras-aseguramiento-salud.aspx

COS: https://www.binasss.sa.cr/ojssalud/index.php/gestion/article/view/177/318

ECU: https://www.pbs.org/frontlineworld/rough/2007/06/ecuador_healthlinks.

html; http://ilo.org/wcmsp5/groups/public/%2D%2D-americas/%2D%2D-ro-lima/%2D%2D-sro-lima/documents/publication/wcms_510914.pdf

MEX: https://www.inegi.org.mx/temas/derechohabiencia/

PER: https://rpmesp.ins.gob.pe/index.php/rpmesp/article/view/3998
URU: https://www.gub.uy/ministerio-salud-publica/tematica/cobertura-poblacional

Sources for Table 2.2, Fig. 2.3 and the following figures

Country	Excess mortality	Excess mortality per	
Argentina[a]	115,416	254	March/20–7/Oct/21
Bolivia	48,378	416	Jan/20–July/21
Brazil	746,715	355	Jan/20–Aug/21
Chile	43,834	231	Jan/20–20/Sept/21
Colombia	163,956	326	Jan/20–5/July/21
Costa Rica[b]	6584	129	March/20–7/Oct/21
Ecuador	75,559	435	Jan/20–20/Sept/21
Mexico	603,507	479	Jan/20–30/Aug/21
Peru	229,863	707	Jan/20–20/Sept/21
Uruguay[c]	6062	174	March/20–7/Oct/21

https://ourworldindata.org/excess-mortality-covid
[a]*https://datosmacro.expansion.com/otros/coronavirus/argentina*
[b]*https://datosmacro.expansion.com/otros/coronavirus/Costa-Rica*
[c]*https://datosmacro.expansion.com/otros/coronavirus/Uruguay*

The indices:

Both are constructed as a simple average of the percentages of the variables considered for each index. The variables not expressed in percentages are converted into these by a simple rule of three. The highest value for each variable is rounded up to set the 100% benchmark, and each country's percentage is then defined according to it.

The following variables are used for each of the indices:

Infrastructure: Number of beds per thousand inhabitants 2017*; 2. Average number of intensive care beds per 100,000 inhabitants*; Number of doctors per thousand inhabitants (2017)*; Number of nurses per thousand inhabitants*; Radiotherapy units per million inhabitants (latest year available)*; Global Health Security Index 2019**; Mechanical ventilators per hundred thousand inhabitants***.

Performance: Percentage of the population vaccinated per year*; Percentage of women examined at least four times during pregnancy*; Maternal mortality rate per 100,000 births*; Mortality in children under five per 1000 births*; Cancer Preparedness Index*

*OECD, World Bank Group (2020), "Health at a Glance: Latin America and the Caribbean 2020", OECD Publishing, París, https://www.oecd-ilibrary.org/sites/6089164f-en/index.html?itemId=/content/publication/6089164f-en;

**2019 Global Health Index, https://www.ghsindex.org/;

***Global Health Intelligence (2020), "Infografia sobre el nivel de preparación de hospitales latinoamericanos ante coronavirus",

****World Cancer Initiative (2020), "Preparación para el abordaje del cáncer en América Latina", https://www.iccp-portal.org/system/files/resources/PREPARACION_PARA_ABORDAJE_CANCER_AMERICA_LATINA.pdf

References

AFP. (2020, May 03). Jair Bolsonaro se rebela contra confinamiento mientras que Brasil registra 100,000 casos de COVID-19. *El Economista*. Accessed February 25, 2025, from https://www.eleconomista.com.mx/internacionales/Jair-Bolsonaro-se-rebela-contra-confinamiento-mientras-que-Brasil-registra-100000-casos-de-Covid-19-20200503-0039.html

Alvarado, C. (2020, July 12). Discurso completo del presidente Carlos Alvarado en cadena Nacional. *Elmundo.cr.* Accessed February 25, 2025, from https://elmundo.cr/costa-rica/discurso-completo-del-presidente-carlos-alvarado-en-cadena-nacional

Arendt, H. (1954). On authority. In *Between past and future*.

Arrossi, S., et al. (2008). Social inequality in Pap smear coverage: Identifying under-users of cervical cancer screening in Argentina. *Reproductive Health Matters, 16*(32), 50–58.

Arroyo-Laguna, J. (2023). ≤Sistemas de salud resilientes para países ya resilientes? Los discursos de la pandemia en la era post COVID-19. *Ciência & Saúde Coletiva*.

Badillo, D. (2020, March 21). AMLO y sus polémicas declaraciones sobre el coronavirus. *El Economista*. Accessed March 11, 2025, from https://www.eleconomista.com.mx/politica/AMLO-y-sus-polemicas-declaraciones-sobre-el-coronavirus-20200321-0001.html

Barbosa, E. C., & Cookson, R. (2019). Multiple inequities in health care: An example from Brazil. *Social Science & Medicine, 228*, 1–8.

Bensusán, G. (in press). La interacción entre políticas laborales y sociales ante la pandemia: Coaliciones sociopolíticas y trayectorias institucionales en cuatro países de la región. In I. Bizberg (Coord.), *Diversidad de Capitalismos: Del auge de las materias primas a la pandemia*. CLACSO.

Bizberg, I., (2021). Politics and the pandemic," Interventions Économiques. Papers in Political Economy, Hors Série. Transformations.

Bizberg, I. (2022). "Latin American Health Regimes in the Face of the Pandemic," Interventions Économiques. Papers in Political Economy, no. 67.

Bizberg, I. (2024). *Four worlds of the welfare state in Latin America*. Palgrave-Macmillan.

Comisión Económica para América Latina y el Caribe (CEPAL). (2021). *Estudio económico de América Latina y el Caribe, 2021* (LC/PUB.2021/10-P/Rev.1). Santiago.

ECLAC. (2021). *Preliminary overview of the economies of Latin America and the Caribbean (2020)*. United Nations.

Evans, P. (1995). *Embedded autonomy: States and industrial transformation*. Princeton University Press.

Figueiredo Santos, J. A. (2018). Classe social, território e desigualdade de saúde no Brasil. *Saúde Soc., 27*(2), 556–572.

Fernández, A. (2020). Alberto Fernández sobre el coronavirus y la economía: "No estamos aquí para dejar caer empresas y argentinos sin trabajo". Accessed October 18, 2024, from https://www.pagina12.com.ar/259840-alberto-fernandez-sobre-el-coronavirus-y-la-economia-no-esta

Galarraga Gortázar, N. (2020, April 16). Bolsonaro destituye al ministro de Salud en plena crisis del coronavirus. *El País*. Accessed February 25, 2025, from https://elpais.com/internacional/2020-04-16/el-ministro-de-salud-de-brasil-afirma-que-el-presidente-bolsonaro-lo-ha-destituido.html

Galindo, J. (2020, March 18). El descrédito populista. *El País*.

García-Subirats, I., et al. (2014). Determinantes del uso de distintos niveles asistenciales en el Sistema General de Seguridad Social en Salud y Sistema Único de Salud en Colombia y Brasil. *Gaceta Sanitaria, 28*(6), 480–488.
Gragnolati, M., Lindelow, M., & Couttolenc, B. (2013). *Twenty years of health system reform in Brazil: An assessment of the Sistema Único de Saúde*. Directions in Development. World Bank.
Han, B.-C. (2020, February 21). La emergencia viral y el mundo de mañana. *El País*. https://elpais.com/ideas/2020-03-21/la-emergencia-viral-y-el-mundo-de-manana-byung-chul-han-el-filosofo-surcoreano-que-piensa-desde-berlin.html
Jassanoff, S., et al. (2021). *Comparative Covid response: Crisis, knowledge, politics interim report*. Harvard Kennedy School.
Kurtz, M. J. (2013). *Social foundations of institutional order* (pp. 66–94). Cambridge University Press. (Kindle version).
Lacalle Pou, L. (2020, July 15). Luis Lacalle Pou, anti-cuarentena: « No estaba dispusesto a ir rumbo a un estadopoliciaco". *Perfil*. Accessed February 25, 2025.
Mann, M. (1984). The autonomous power of the state: Its origins, mechanisms, and results. *European Journal of Sociology / Archives Européennes de Sociologie / Europäisches Archiv für Soziologie, 25*(2), 185–213.
Mesa-Lago, C. (1994). *Changing social security in Latin America: Towards alleviating the social costs of economic reform*. Lynne Rienner Publishers.
Nuñez, A., & Chi, C. (2013). Equity in health utilization in Chile. *International Journal for Equity in Health, 12*(58), 1–16.
Our World in Data. (2024). *Coronavirus (COVID-19) data*. Our World in Data. https://ourworldindata.org/coronavirus
Palacios, A., Espinola, N., & Rojas-Roque, C. (2020). Need and inequality in the use of health care services in a fragmented and decentralized health system: Evidence for Argentina. *International Journal for Equity in Health, 19*(67), 1–14.
Piñera, S. (2020, March 13). Presidente Piñera anuncia medidas por Coronavirus. *Gobierno de Chile*. https://prensa.presidencia.cl/discurso.aspx?id=138176
Ruiz Gómez, F., Zapata Jaramillo, T., & Garavito Beltrán, L. (2013). Colombian health care system: Results on equity for five health dimensions, 2003–2008. *Revista Panamericana de Salud Pública, 33*(2), 107–115.
Sánchez-Talanquer, M., et al. (2020). *La respuesta de México al COVID: Estudio de caso*. Institute for Global Health Sciences, UCSF.
Soifer, H. D. (2015). *State building in Latin America*. Cambridge University Press.
Schneider, E. C., Sarnak, D. O., Squires, D., Shah, A., & Doty, M. M. (2017). *Mirror, mirror 2017: International comparison reflects flaws and opportunities for better U.S. health care*. Commonwealth Fund.
Tikkanen, R., et al. (2020). *International profiles of health care systems*. The Commonwealth Fund. https://www.commonwealthfund.org/sites/default/files/2020-12/International_Profiles_of_Health_Care_Systems_Dec2020.pdf
Tocqueville, A. (1981). *De la Démocratie en Amérique*. Garnier-Flammarion.
Vasquez, F., Paraje, G., & Estay, M. (2013). Income-related inequality in health and health care utilization in Chile, 2000–2009. *Revista Panamericana de Salud Pública, 33*(2), 98–106.

Chapter 3
Tracing Test Capacity in Latin America During the COVID-19 Pandemic

Isamu Okada

3.1 Introduction

"We have a simple message to all countries: test, test, test," the Director General of WHO announced in a press conference on March 16, 2020 (Farge & Revill, 2020). Scaling up the test capacity became a part of the standard policy package for designing policies that pursue maximum health safety with minimum social costs. In the implementation phase, however, the responses across countries differed in the following months (Capano et al., 2020). In the current literature, the direct effect of test capacity on health outcomes is unclear[1] and underexplored. One reason for this under-exploration is the limited empirical data of the actual test performance. This chapter tries to fill this critical void with daily survey data collected through Facebook and shared by the University of Maryland. The data enables us to visualize how the COVID-19 tests varied across countries and over time from the viewpoint of survey participants.

This chapter identifies the test capacity limitation and uses Latin American countries for illustration. To be precise, it examines issues in the measurement of test capacity. While true test counts are not clear from official data, I expand data options and propose alternative measurement ideas. I also assess what aspect of state capacity the test capacity elucidates and how it may link with a notable health outcome,

[1] Rannan-Eliya et al. (2021) claim that an increase in TCR test-to-case ratio (TCR) as a proxy of testing intensity reduces the effective reproduction number. This study seems to have a technical problem. Because the test-to-case ratio takes infected cases as the denominator, the ratio becomes smaller as the infected cases decrease. At the same time, the effective reproduction number should also take a smaller value as cases decrease.

I. Okada (✉)
Nagoya University, Nagoya, Japan
e-mail: okada.isamu.w8@f.mail.nagoya-u.ac.jp

I. Okada (ed.), *COVID-19 and State Capacity in Latin America*, Latin American Societies, https://doi.org/10.1007/978-3-032-15572-6_3

namely, case fatality rate (CFR). Some literature has claimed that state capacity effectively mitigates the health risk derived from COVID-19 infection (Alfano & Ercolano, 2022; Bosancianu et al., 2020; Gisselquist & Vaccaro, 2023; Serikbayeva et al., 2021). Yet, they used generic pre-pandemic measurements such as Worldwide Governance Indicators (WGI) and Fragile State Index (FSI). As a more nuanced alternative, this chapter deploys specific measurements on test capacity from daily survey data and demonstrates how it updates our understanding of the state capacity puzzle. To illustrate multi-channeled and configurational effects, I use fuzzy-set qualitative comparative analysis (QCA).

I selected Latin American countries and a specific period from June to December 2020 to enhance the validation of the proposed measurement with context specificity (Adcock & Collier, 2001). Measurements become more trustworthy if they are congruent with other referential indexes. The comparison within Latin America can provide an illustration that is comparable with previous discussions on early state responses to the pandemic and other related literature on state capacity in the region (Brinks et al., 2020; Kurtz, 2013; Saylor, 2014; Soifer, 2015). I set my scope on the 6 months from June to December 2020, excluding the first few months in 2020 when haphazard reactions and irregularities were likely to overwhelm systematic trends, and the later period from 2021 when the availability of vaccines transformed the landscape and the meaning of testing.

The following parts are divided into four sections. Section 3.2 provides the theoretical framework on the related topic and clarifies gaps in the previous knowledge. Section 3.3 describes the data retrieved from the project of Meta and the University of Maryland and, briefly, the Latin American case. Section 3.4 reports empirical analyses and results, and Sect. 3.5 concludes.

3.2 Theory

3.2.1 Test Capacity as a State Capacity

State capacity for the pandemic responses includes hard and soft resources in health care systems and the whole gamut of public administration infrastructure that enables the appropriate design and implementation of policies for mitigating health risk and other associated costs. State capacity literature has focused on "legibility," or the capacity of the state to collect high-quality information through census, civil registration, and other statistics (Brambor et al., 2020; Lee & Zhang, 2017; Scott, 2008). Under this logic, COVID-19 test capacity is a quintessential example that speaks to the capacity of the state to collect information for designing and implementing policy measures at a time of crisis. Beyond the epistemological interest, variations in test capacity inform the contemporary outlook of state capacity that is projected by a common exogenous shock (Capano, 2020; Capano et al., 2020).

All COVID-19 tests are purported to provide a picture of infection spread as clearly as possible, even though there are different types of tests: molecular assays like Polymerase Chain Reaction (PCR), antigen tests, and serological (antibody) tests (Mercer & Salit, 2021). PCR has the highest accuracy[2] and can detect infections even for asymptomatic and pre-symptomatic patients. It is relatively expensive, however, and the speed of assays may highly depend on the available facilities and human resources. Antigen tests can be much quicker and may have advantages in quick diagnosis and scaling up the test capacity within a limited time scope (Peeling et al., 2021). This, however, tends to have lower accuracy and increase false negatives for asymptomatic and pre-symptomatic patients (Scohy et al., 2020). Serological tests detect antibodies that signal the infection experience of a person to SARS-CoV-19 in the past, but it tends to lack sensitivity to pre-symptomatic or asymptomatic cases with recent infection. It may also report false positives from infections in the not-recent past and coronaviruses other than SARS-CoV-19.

Regardless of the test variation, overall test capacity provides a baseline for other capacity items that provide more direct consequences on the spread of COVID-19 infection (Cheng et al., 2020; Mercer & Salit, 2021). Tests are used to detect SARS-CoV-19 infection, which establishes a precise diagnosis to decide on proper healthcare treatments. In addition, the identification of the virus in symptomatic, asymptomatic, and pre-symptomatic persons enables contact tracing that preempts or contains outbreaks at a community level. Tests can be employed at specific spots or categories of people (e.g., airports, residential districts, classrooms, randomly sampled populations) for surveillance and forming adaptive policy decisions. Massive population-scale tests provide an empirical basis for designing policies to reduce effective reproduction numbers (Pollán et al., 2020). In a nutshell, if test capacity is limited, it would likely result not only in underestimating infection spreading but also in constraining other infection-containing measures.

3.2.2 *What Test Capacity Limitations Mean*

What kind of gaps are limitations in test capacity? Test schemes depend on the available resources and adopted policies. Following Brinks et al. (2020), I formulate the limitation in test capacity by three items, namely, the baseline status (S_0), the desirable achievement (S'), and the actual achievement (S). The limitation is the gap between what should be achieved ($S' - S_0$) and what was achieved ($S - S_0$).

I assume the same S_0 and S' for all countries and hence consider that capacity limitation is the gap in what was achieved ($S - S_0$). S_0 must be equally set as no states in the world were implementing COVID-19 testing by the end of 2019. A few East Asian countries that suffered from the SARS outbreak in 2003 had

[2] Technically, sensitivity refers to the correct identification of positive infection and specificity to that of negative cases (Mercer & Salit, 2021). Otherwise clearly indicated, I use accuracy to mean either or both of these two terms.

better-prepared systems for scaling up test capacity (An & Tang, 2020); this is not the baseline difference but a part of the capacity. I also assume that the desirable testing scale (S') is the same for all countries and should not be confused with such visions proclaimed by political leaders (Aruguete et al., 2021; Gramacho & Turgeon, 2021; Jarquin & Marti i Puig, 2021; Medeiros et al., 2021). Policies might shape policy goals—strategic resource allocation, political ideology, or other reasons—but cannot define what scale of tests a country ultimately needs to satisfy the necessary conditions for whatever policies follow.

What factors affect test capacity? Although I don't examine this question as a main focus of this chapter, it is useful to look up the factors for envisioning when and under what conditions test capacity tends to appear limited. Aside from the political factors discussed previously, I assume available resources and their allocation as the most crucial reasons. Limited test capacity can be due to shortcomings in public health resources. Test capacity is determined by laboratory capacity, the availability of equipment and human resources, and the budget for scaling them up in the short run (Benítez et al., 2020). Latin American countries suffered low health equipment supplies from the domestic industry in the first year, and the shortcomings were exacerbated by global export restrictions (CEPAL, 2020). In Peru, antigen and antibody tests were the most used during the early time due to missing laboratories for PCRs (Delgado-Diaz et al., 2021). Beyond the public domain, increasing test capacity in a short period needed the involvement of public and private institutions (Cyr et al., 2021; Kameda et al., 2021). Uruguay outperformed in the "testing war" thanks to public–private collaborations and test system decentralization (Taylor, 2020). Another related factor is the financial cost required for citizens who want to test. Trudeau et al. (2020) confirm economic cost as a crucial factor for people opting out from receiving tests.

What consequences would test capacity limitations produce? As mentioned, an immediate consequence is the underestimation of infection cases and deaths related to COVID-19 and potentially inaccurate diagnoses. Another consequence, in the medium rather than short term, is the challenge in infection containment elaboration due to the lack of accurate information on infection spreading.

3.2.3 Limitations in the Knowledge of Capacity Limitations

A primary challenge in the previous literature is empirical. Previous studies used Government Effectiveness in Worldwide Governance Indicators (WGI) (Serikbayeva et al., 2021) and the Fragile State Index (FSI) (Gisselquist & Vaccaro, 2023), to argue the causal linkage between state capacity in general and COVID-19 mortality. However, these are generic and do not specifically target health-related capacities. Others used health expenditures and the number of medical doctors and ICU beds (González-Bustamante, 2021; Schaefer et al., 2020). Although certainly related to the health sector, these may not necessarily reflect the test capacity.

The foremost challenge is incomplete information in the official record of test counts. Figure 3.1 illustrates the daily report and smoothed number of tests per thousand population from Our World in Data (OWiD). The information for Honduras, Nicaragua, and Venezuela is missing due to inaccessibility of official or other sources in the original data. Peru only reported the cumulative numbers. In addition, irregular fluctuations at specific time points in Brazil and El Salvador suggest inaccuracy in their daily updates.

Against this backdrop, I contribute to two major fronts. First, I provide an alternative measurement for state capacity from the daily COVID-19 Trends and Impact Survey (CTIS) data collected via Facebook by the University of Maryland and Meta. This data source enables us to capture the testing capacity limitations by shifting the approach from state-originated information—which is endogenous to the very state capacity—to self-report by ordinary citizens. Using the CTIS data may still contain other measurement problems. Test-taking experience can be conditioned by (a) the reasons to take a test and (b) the reasons to participate in a voluntary survey related to the pandemic. To circumvent this problem, I focus on specific gaps in testing experience trends over 6 months from June to December 2020. My second contribution is to probe the linkage between test capacity limitations and health outcomes, such as positive cases and mortality due to COVID-19. I examine how much our understanding can be upgraded thanks to test capacity measurements from CTIS data. Assuming the possibility that test capacity and other state capacities each have effects through different channels on the health outcome, I examine configurational causal pathways with fuzzy-set QCA.

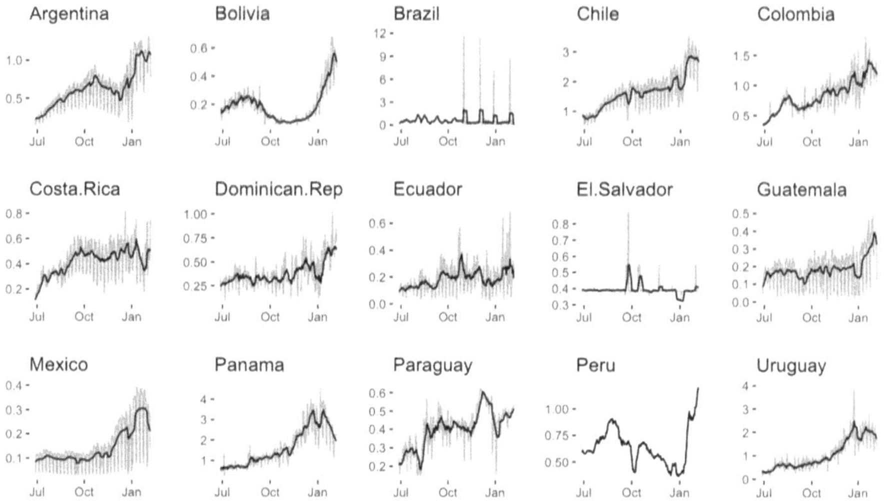

Fig. 3.1 Official test counts (gray) and the smoothed lines (black) in Latin American countries. Daily test counts are missing for Peru in the original data. Source: Hasell et al. (2020); the dataset was retrieved from https://ourworldindata.org/coronavirus-testing (last access June 16, 2023)

3.3 The Case and Data

Before proceeding to empirical analysis, I briefly explain the CTIS data and the Latin American context. In general, state capacity limitations start with incomplete data accessibility in the official source, and therefore it is not a surprise that scholars use alternative resources like surveys (Luna & Soifer, 2017). This societal approach was also adopted by burgeoning studies of the pandemic that use survey data collected through social media or online platforms (Alicea-Planas et al., 2021; Aruguete et al., 2021; Calvo & Ventura, 2021; Piazza & Schwier, 2021; Urrunaga-Pastor et al., 2021).

I use the CTIS data to fill the void in accessing test capacity limitations. The CTIS extended all over the world largely from late April 2020, recruiting survey participants through direct invitations on Facebook walls. The participation was voluntary on an opt-in basis, and the questionnaire was slightly modified along the way.[3] I focus on the period from June 27 to December 27, 2020, for certain reasons. First, I excluded the first 3 months from the WHO declaration of the global pandemic, suspecting that this period informs more about accidental irregularities than systemic patterns. I also excluded the period when vaccines started to be available. Second, the CTIS data that I will extensively use changed the questionnaire design over time, and the questions of my interest were incorporated only from June 27, 2020. Also, the survey collected an extraordinarily large sample size from December 28 to 30 in most target countries compared to previous days, so I decided to exclude the period from December 28, 2020.

Latin American countries provide a good number of comparable cases with salient damages caused by the pandemic. Also, the region has contributed to the rich debate on state capacity, especially by the renowned fact that its cross-national ranking remained mostly unchanged for more than a century (Kurtz, 2013; Mahoney, 2010; Soifer, 2015; Yashar, 2018), which enables us to be cautious of unrealistic findings that might occur from complex data operationalization.

During the target period, Latin American countries exhibited remarkable variations. Most countries experienced the first wave of the COVID-19 outbreak, which caused 100–300 daily reported cases (Fig. 3.2). The wave peaks differed; for instance, Chile was coming to the end of the first wave at the beginning of the period, while Uruguay faced its first wave much later. Many countries suffered a rapid increase in cases in the middle of this period. Most countries maintained a series of stringent controls on social activities, except for Nicaragua and Uruguay, and were on the way to liberating social contacts throughout the period (S3.3 Fig. in Supplementary Files).

[3] The sample size for each country and its time-series variation is cataloged in S3.1 Table and S3.2 Fig. in Supplementary Files. Although voluntary participation via Facebook may share specific characteristics not common to the whole population (Castorena et al., 2023), this data collection is a crucial supply that complements the given data shortage. I will discuss some limitations in the last section.

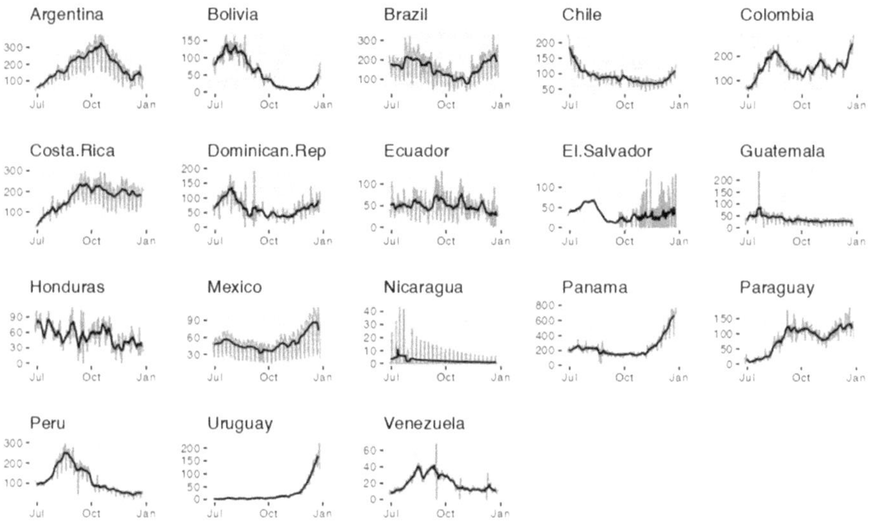

Fig. 3.2 Daily reported cases per million population (gray) and its 7-day moving average (black). Source: Our World in Data, https://ourworldindata.org/covid-cases (last access, June 30, 2023)

The countries were also dissimilar in their test policies (S3.4 Fig.) and contact tracing policies (S3.5 Fig.). We can notice three groups in terms of test policies. The first group applied open public testing, fully or partially, over the target period. Uruguay is an outlier having this policy throughout the period, and Chile, Panama, Peru, and Venezuela applied this for a part of the period. The second group applied tests to anyone with COVID-19 symptoms. Argentina, Brazil, Chile, Colombia, Dominican Republic, Ecuador, Guatemala, Panama, and Peru followed this pattern for most of the period. The third group focused on testing people who met certain criteria and with symptoms. This last category includes Bolivia, Costa Rica, El Salvador, Honduras, Mexico, Nicaragua, and Paraguay. Regarding contact tracing policies, Argentina, Brazil, Chile, Colombia, Panama, Paraguay, and Peru tried to apply comprehensive contact tracing. Meanwhile, no such policy was adopted by Nicaragua and Venezuela, and other countries applied it to a part of the infected cases.

3.4 Empirical Analysis

3.4.1 Identifying Test Capacity Limitations

The CTIS reports the daily counts of tested people (Fig. 3.3). But, this indicator is a mixed product of test capacity, test policy, and infection trends, which cannot be easily separated from one another. The 7-day moving average in tested informants started from around 50% at the end of June 2020 and went into decline in almost all

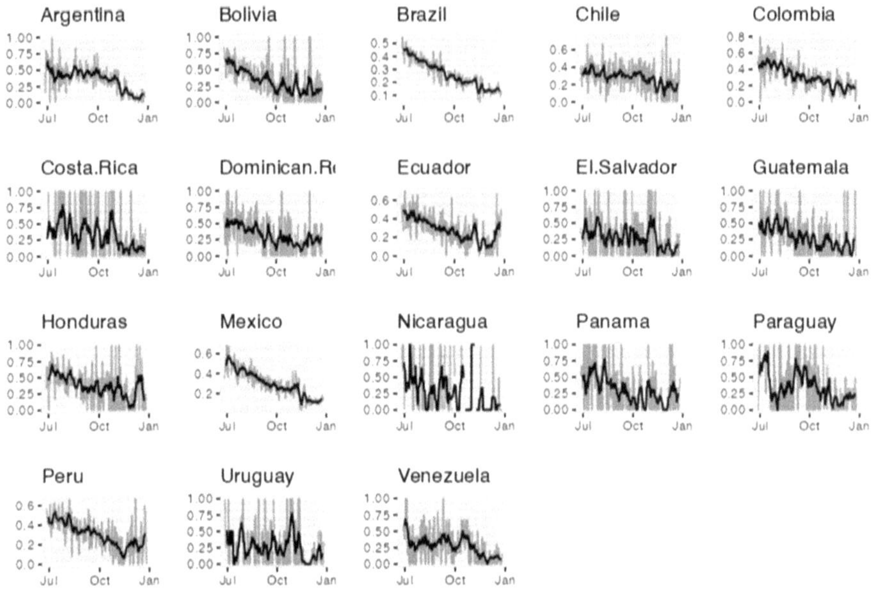

Fig. 3.3 The percentage of tested persons (gray) and 7-day moving average (black). Source: CTIS data

countries. This can be due to declining infection trends—and fewer people worried about testing—or dwindling test capacity due to limited test kits supply in the surging infection numbers. It can also be due to different test policies and their changes over time, which create diverging trends across countries and further complicate our interpretation.

Instead, I use the gap between demand and supply for test service provision as a measurement that addresses the test capacity limitations. The CTIS asked participants if they had taken a test or not in the past 14 days. It also asked if they wanted to take one in case they answered not being tested. Taking advantage of these data and calculating the gap between the actual test experience and the unmet demand is a more reliable source since the baseline is the people's demand for tests, which is supposed to control the infection trend on the ground and what people expect in the given local environment of test policy. The broader and faster the infection spreads from the viewpoint of survey participants, the more they would demand tests, and test policy should accompany it regardless of whatever excuse. If infection trends calm down, the number of people demanding tests would decline too, but the gap in test implementation would remain for those who still need it. Figure 3.4 reports the time-series changes in the percentage of "not-tested-but-wanted" people among the survey participants and its 7-day moving average. The 7-day average is almost constant over the 6-month period.

Based on this data, I crafted two indicators that represent test capacity limitations. I denominate the first as the *non-tested ratio*, that is the not-tested-but-wanted

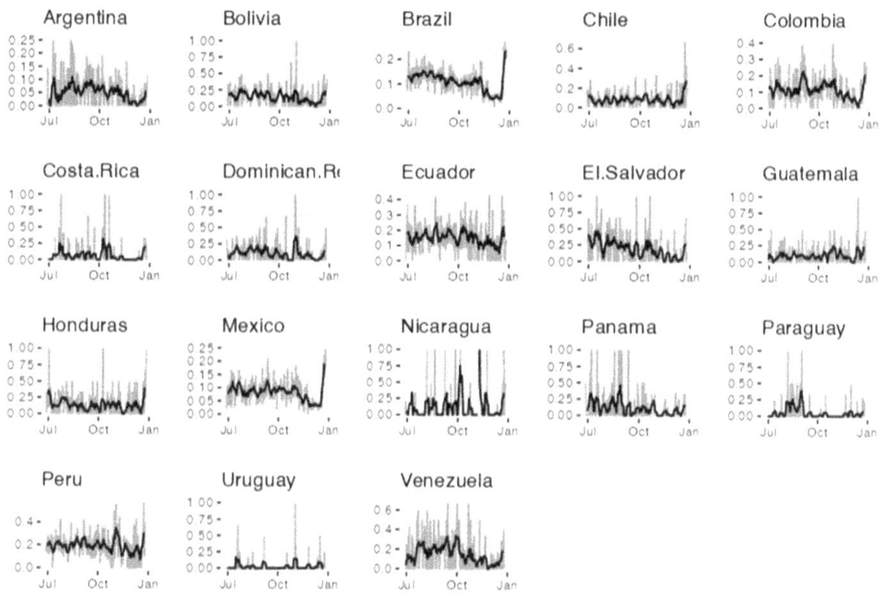

Fig. 3.4 The percentage of "not-tested-but-wanted" people (gray) and 7-day moving average (black). Source: CTIS data

people's percentage among those who wanted a test—the sum of non-tested and tested people— and the second as the *non-tested percentage*, that is the not-tested-but-wanted people's percentage among all survey participants. I use two indicators to avoid measurement errors potentially caused by the limited sample size in some selected countries (n = min. 229 ~ max. 22,857). Then, I take each country's mean score for each indicator for 6 months from June 27 to December 27, 2020, to mitigate the problem caused by the same sample size limitation. S3.6 Fig. in Supplementary File illustrates the relationship between these two indicators.

3.4.2 Test Capacity Limitations and Other Indicators

How well do the two indicators represent actual test capacity limitations? While there are no direct ways to determine their validity, I check them through some assumptions. First, I expect that the *non-tested ratio* and *percentage* would overlap with the general indicators of state capacity to some extent, as both speak to governmental effectiveness. Second, I expect the two indicators to covary with health expenditure available in each country since how quickly and sufficiently test kits are supplied is assumed to be related to available budgets. Yet, as I argued, test capacity should not perfectly correlate with the other indicators. Test capacity is more a question of the extensive reach of test kits and specific laboratories for diagnosis than other general issues. Also, budget sizes alone cannot explain test capacity limitations.

Figures 3.5 and 3.6 illustrate how the *non-tested ratio* and *percentage* are related to other available indicators such as the Fragile State Index (FSI), Government Effectiveness (WGI), and health expenditure in 2019. The correlation is remarkably high with all the indicators, suggesting that *non-tested ratios* and *percentages* are by and large related to the relative volume of health expenditure and referential scores of state capacity in other data sources. Still, a few outliers are notable. Peru (PER) and El Salvador (SLV) demonstrate considerably higher test capacity limitations as compared with baseline state capacity suggested by the FSI and WGI scores (Fig. 3.5) and health expenditure (Fig. 3.6). In contrast, Paraguay reported remarkably lower test capacity limitations even though its FSI and WGI scores and health expenditure were similar to El Salvador. Overall, my measurements for test capacity limitations sketch a similar trend as depicted by conventional state capacity indicators with a few exceptions.

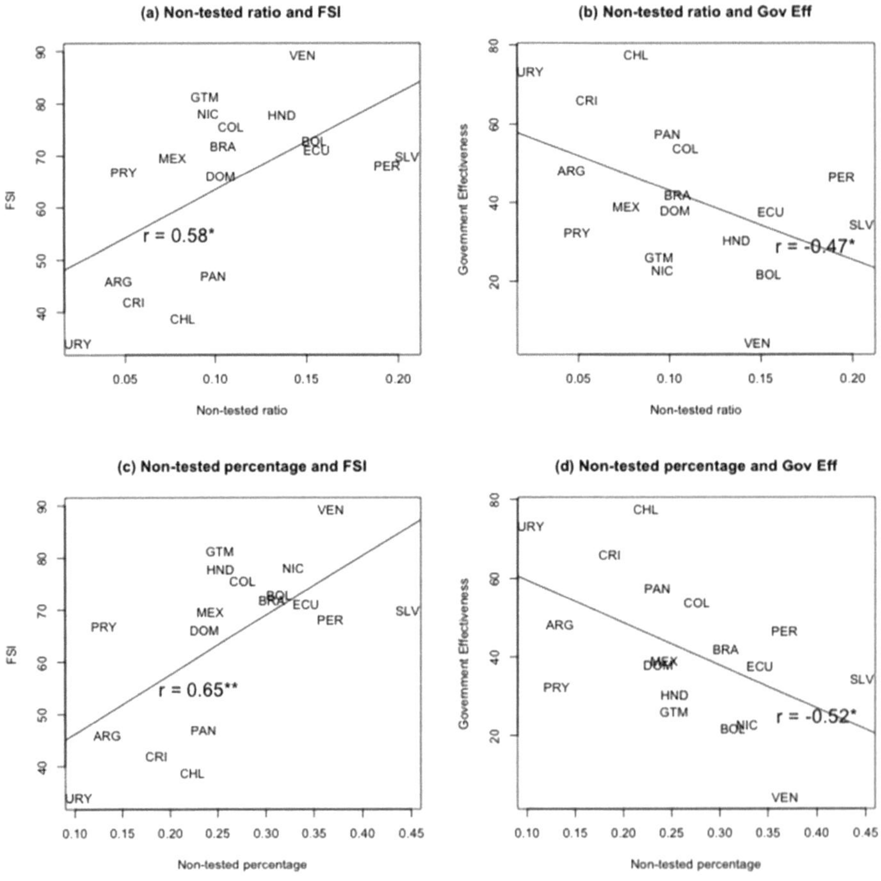

Fig. 3.5 Test limitations and state capacity index. *p < 0.05, **p < 0.01. Source: Author

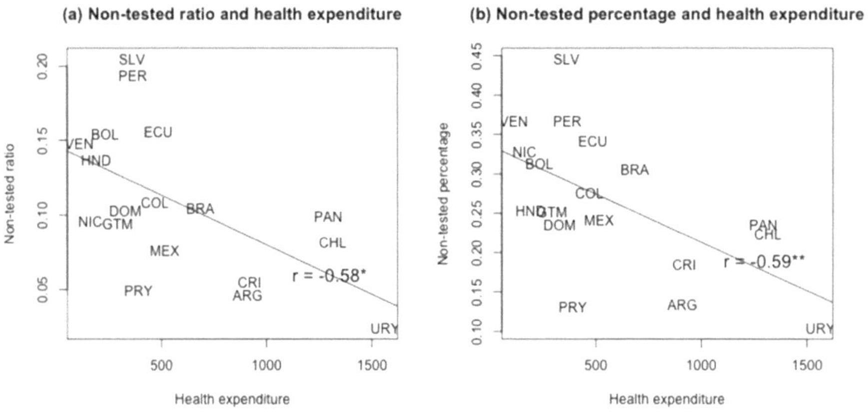

Fig. 3.6 Test limitations and health expenditure. *p < 0.05, **p < 0.01. Source: Author

3.4.3 Test Capacity Limitations and Reported Cases

How much can test capacity limitations explain health outcomes? As with the other ways to check the validity of the *non-tested ratios* and *percentages*, I revisit how much these indicators can explain the available health outcome scores: reported infection cases and case fatality rates. I examine them in order in this and the following subsections.

The relationship between test capacity limitations and the infection cases reported is not simple. I assume test capacity limitations have two distinctive causal mechanisms, and both are conditioned by general state capacity. The first mechanism suggests that higher test capacity limitations result in underestimating the magnitude of infected cases. According to this assumption, the higher *non-tested ratios* and *percentages* should coincide with the lower cases reported. On the contrary, the second mechanism considers that lower test capacity is related to a larger number of cases since test capacity limitations may lead to lower capacity to design and implement infection-containing measures such as contact tracing and vice versa. Hence, the higher *non-tested ratios* and *percentages* should report higher cases. The distinction between the two mechanisms is the general state capacity—beyond test capacity per se—since the underestimation of infected cases is likely because of a baseline institutional weakness, while the infection-containing measures require a general institutional strength.

Table 3.1 summarizes my assumption. If both general state capacity and test capacity are limited, we should witness a small number of cases because of underestimation. If a country has a high general capacity and not limited test capacity (a lower *non-tested ratio* and *percentage*), I expect a large or small number of cases because the effectiveness of infection containment may hinge on other capacities relative to the design and implementation of infection-containing measures. I hold no assumptions for the other two scenarios.

Table 3.1 Assumptions on test capacity limitations and cases reported

		Test capacity	
		Not limited (lower *non-tested ratio* and *percentage*)	Limited (higher *non-tested ratio* and *percentage*)
General state capacity	High	A large number of cases (correct report) or A small number of cases (containment success)	No assumption
	Low	No assumption	A small number of cases (underestimation)

Source: Author

The findings corroborate my assumption. In Fig. 3.7, countries with higher general state capacity, higher than 39 for WGI (median = 38.58) and lower than 70 for FSI scores (median = 69.75), respectively, are indicated in black, and otherwise in gray. I focus on the countries with higher *non-tested ratios* and *percentage*s (at the right end of each Fig.: Peru, Bolivia, Ecuador, Honduras, El Salvador, and Venezuela) and that with the lower scores (at the left end: Argentina, Costa Rica, and Uruguay). On the one hand, countries with high general state capacity and lower *non-tested ratios* and *percentages* are reported with a large number of cases (Argentina, Costa Rica, and Panama) or a small number of cases (Uruguay). This matches the common appraisal that Uruguay succeeded in containing virus spreading even though maintaining less stringent measures during most of 2020 (Bidegain et al., 2021; Taylor, 2020).

On the other hand, countries with *low* general capacity and certain test capacity limitations are reported with small numbers of cases (Bolivia, Ecuador, El Salvador, Honduras, and Venezuela). In contrast, Peru, which has *high* general capacity and high test capacity limitation, reported a larger number of cases per million compared to these other countries in the group of higher *non-tested ratios* and *percentages*. There is a possibility of underestimation as suggested for the former group, echoing the literature on Venezuela (Paniz-Mondolfi et al., 2020) and two Central American peers (Pearson et al., 2021).

3.4.4 Test Capacity Limitations and Case Fatality Rates

Previous literature has argued that general state capacity, as measured by the FSI and WGI, reduces case fatality rates (CFR), which is the number of COVID-19 deaths divided by the reported cases (Bosancianu et al., 2020; Gisselquist & Vaccaro, 2023; Serikbayeva et al., 2021). I revisit this claim and examine how test capacity limitations upgrade it. Due to the small sample size (n = 18), I cannot apply the same statistical methods as the previous literature. Instead, I use fuzzy-set QCA to corroborate the relationships between my test capacity indicators, general state capacity indicators, and other factors. This methodological choice is also reliable

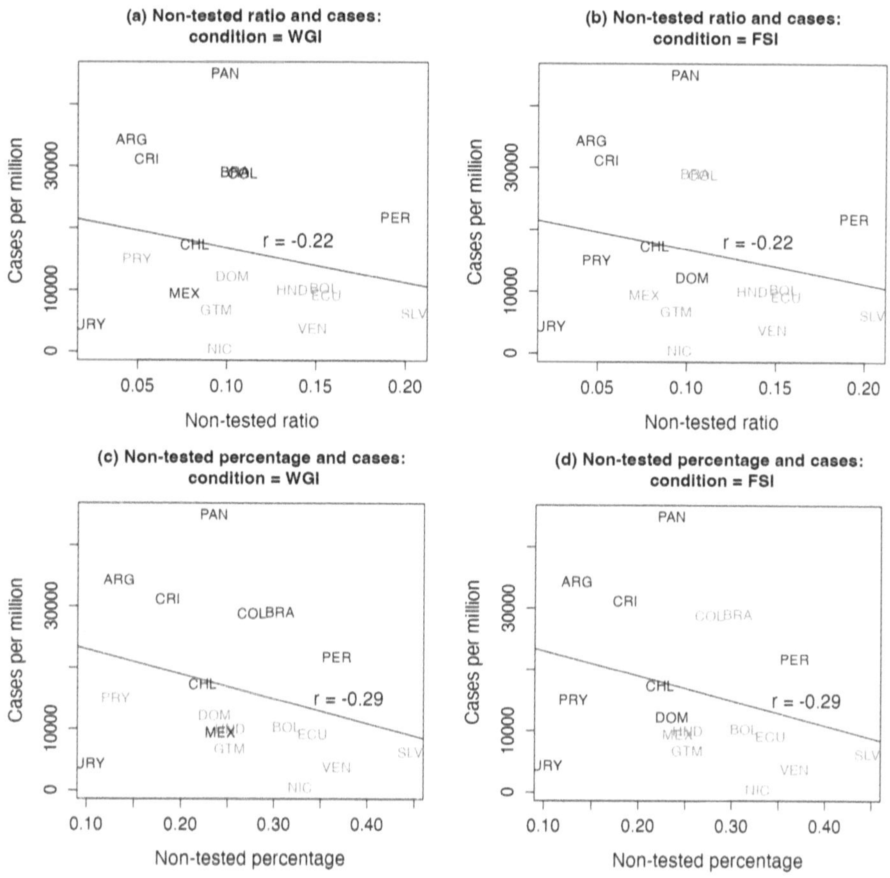

Fig. 3.7 Test limitations and cases reported. Countries with WGI higher than 38 and FSI scores lower than 69 are indicated in black and otherwise in gray. No correlation index was higher than the 95% statistical significance level. Source: Author

because causal mechanisms about test capacity and general state capacity can be multifold and independent of each other.

Qualitative Comparative Analysis (QCA) examines how much the presence or absence of the conditions (independent variables) coincides with the presence or absence of the outcome (dependent variable) (Schneider & Wagemann, 2012). Different from statistical estimation techniques, it takes configurational causal assumptions, assuming the presence and absence of the same condition as asymmetrical, the combined effects of two or more conditions as common, and multiple causal pathways that connect different sets of conditions to the outcome without difficulty. Fuzzy-set QCA allows researchers to calibrate variables beyond the simplest binary—presence or absence—set-theoretical assumption by assigning fuzzy scores, which are continuous values that range from 0 to 1 (Ragin, 2008). The

Table 3.2 Calibration

	Full membership	Cut-off	Full non-membership
Outcome			
CFR	0.005	0.05	0.1
Condition			
Non-tested percentage	0.15	0.25	0.3
Non-tested ratio	0.06	0.1	0.13
Few-non-tested	Full membership to Non-tested percentage and (∩) Non-tested ratio = 1, otherwise 0		
FSI	40	60	80
Government effectiveness (WGI)	70	50	30
GovEff-FSI	Full membership to FSI and (∩) Government effectiveness = 1, otherwise 0		
Political regime (FH)	2	1.5	1
Stringency Index (OxCGRT)	80	50	20
Health expenditure (WHO)	900	700	500
Cases per million (OWiD)	30,000	10,000	5000

Source: Author

operationalization and the endpoint explanation require the researcher's reasoning and case-based interpretation.

The outcome of the assessment here is the case fatality rate (CFR). The conditions are the *non-tested ratio* and *percentage*, FSI, Government effectiveness from WGI, political regime status from Freedom House,[4] Stringency Index by Oxford COVID-19 Government Response Tracker (GxCGRT), health expenditure by World Health Organization (WHO), and reported cases per million (OWiD).[5] The conditions and the outcome were calibrated into fuzzy scores by setting full membership, full non-membership, and cut-off (the most ambiguous) points as shown in Table 3.2.[6] Except for the two test capacity indicators, I incorporated those variables used and tested in previous literature. For an easier post-analysis interpretation, I calibrated all variables so that they take full membership for the "desirable" situation; CFR, *non-tested ratio* and *percentage*, and FSI must be smaller, while the rest must be bigger. In order to mitigate the problem of an inflated number of conditions amidst the limited diversity of cases, I crafted two integrated conditions:

[4] Based on the Freedom in the World dataset that combines political rights and civil liberties, I categorized both Free and Partly-Free countries as 1 and Non-Free countries as 0.

[5] CFR, *non-tested ratio*, *non-tested percentage*, and cases per million were calculated for the entire study period (from 6/27/2020 to 12/27/2020). Other conditions took the values in 2019.

[6] I used the directed methods with logistic function based on the distribution of values among countries. I used the package QCA in R. The values for each country and the membership scores are visualized in S3.7 Fig. in Supplementary File.

Few-non-tested for those cases with full membership to both non-tested percentage and non-tested ratio, and GovEff-FSI for those with full membership to both FSI and Government effectiveness.

Fuzzy-set QCA examines how the fuzzy scores for the conditions and the outcome consist of sets and subsets to each other. For instance, if the fuzzy score of a condition is consistently higher than that of the outcome all over the cases, the condition is a superset—hence, a necessary condition—of the outcome's presence. When we notice such consistently overvalued fuzzy scores for a subsample of cases, it means the condition sufficiently explains the subsample. In contrast, if a condition score does not consistently overvalue the outcome score among the whole cases or subsample, a systematic relationship is dubious. Researchers can set a threshold for consistency for making such inferences: 0.8 for this study. Moreover, we can minimize the combination of conditions by assessing the indifferent conditions that happen to be present for the outcome's presence but absent for others.[7] Furthermore, to address the limited variation in the set of given cases, we can use unknown cases as counterfactual references while excluding the inconsistent conditions according to the actual data. I will only show what we call parsimonious solutions, which use the sets of conditions empirically unavailable in the given range of cases—assuming those would produce the expected outcome—and give simpler visions for causality (Baumgartner, 2015) in the following report.[8]

I first tested the necessity conditions in fsQCA by setting the consistency cut-off threshold for inclusion as 0.9 and that for relevance as 0.5 at minimum for all 18 Latin American countries. However, there was no recipe satisfying this condition, particularly for the 0.5 relevance threshold.

Now, we turn to the test for sufficiency. The truth table (see S3.8 in Supplementary Files) informs that, among 12 cases with positive outcomes (lower CFR), 7 cases have the *non-tested percentage* present, or non-tested people lower than 25% of all survey-takers. Meanwhile, FSI and Government Effectiveness appeared positive only in four and five cases, respectively.

I analyzed the sufficiency test using three models (Table 3.3). The first model that uses eight conditions suggests three parsimonious solutions to keep a lower CFR: (1) less stringent measures (Nicaragua and Uruguay), (2) low non-tested percentage with a larger number of infected cases, or (3) lower non-tested ratio and with a smaller number of cases. The difference between (2) and (3) would be due to the elevated non-tested ratio—compared to non-tested percentage—in the countries with many infected cases (see S3.6 in Supplementary Files). Meanwhile, GoEff and FSI don't appear as sufficient conditions.

Model 2 analyzes sufficiency by replacing the non-tested percentage and ratio with few-non-tested, which takes 1 when the country has full membership to both non-tested percentage and ratio. The parsimonious solution in this model suggests

[7] I used the package QCA in R for minimization, particularly CCubes, Quine-McCluskey, and the enhanced Quine-McCluskey methods. The results remained the same regardless of methods.

[8] Complex solutions for Model 1 in Table 3.3 are reported in S3.9 in the Supplementary Files.

Table 3.3 Test for sufficiency: parsimonious solutions

Conditions	inclS	PRI	covS	covU	Cases
Model 1 (FH, Non-tested percentage, Non-tested ratio, GovEff, FSI, Stringency, Health expenditure, Cases)					
~Stringency	0.909	0.808	0.231	0.081	NIC, URY
Non-tested percentage*Cases	0.905	0.874	0.408	0.257	ARG, CHI, CRI, DOM, PAN, PRY
Non-tested ratio*~Cases	0.855	0.756	0.370	0.181	ECU, SLV, HON, VEN
Model 2 (FH, Few-non-tested, GovEff-FSI, Stringency, Health expenditure, Cases)					
~FH	0.903	0.856	0.169	0.153	NIC, VEN
Few-non-tested	0.868	0.848	0.207	0.065	ARG, PRY, URY
Health expenditure	0.898	0.877	0.394	0.245	ARG, CHI, CRI, PAN, URY
Model 3 (FH, Few-non-tested, GovEff, FSI, Stringency, Health expenditure, Cases)					
~FH	0.903	0.856	0.169	0.127	NIC, VEN
Few-non-tested	0.868	0.848	0.207	0.048	ARG, PRY, URY
+ Any of the following					
FSI	0.910	0.874	0.471	0.055	ARG, CHI, CRI, PAN, URY
Health expenditure	0.898	0.877	0.394	0.025	ARG, CHI, CRI, PAN, URY

Source: Author
* logical multiplication, ~ the condition's absence

three causal recipes: (1) political regimes with low freedom, (2) few non-tested percentage and ratio, or (3) large health expenditure. Again, government effectiveness and FSI did not show as explanatory of the positive outcome. Model 3 uses the few-non-tested condition and government effectiveness and FSI separately. In this model, parsimonious solutions are (1) low freedom regimes, (2) few non-tested percentage and ratio, or (3) any of low Fragile State Index or large health expenditure.

The series of results suggests that test capacity has a stronger explanatory power compared to FSI and WGI scores. Notably, by closely observing the cases explained by each recipe, we notice that a higher test capacity, either represented by non-tested percentage or ratio, explains 10 countries among 18.

3.5 Conclusion

This study aims to refresh our attention on test capacity limitations under the COVID-19 pandemic, using Latin American countries that scored the severest damages in the first year. Taking advantage of the daily CTIS data, the proposed measurements fill the void of data shortage and other associated problems in the measurement of state capacity, which are usually unavoidable when relying solely on governmental sources. The two test capacity indicators that count the percentage and ratio of non-tested people exhibit gaps in the supply and demand of tests straightforwardly and highlight areas of limited legibility during the COVID-19 pandemic. The two measurements disclose where reported cases of COVID-19 can be underestimated and how broadly the linkage between capacity weaknesses and life risk outcomes can apply beyond the conventional and generic measurements.

The overall analyses present interesting findings, although with some caution for careful interpretation. The reliance on survey-based information is not free from sampling bias and representativeness concerns (Castorena et al., 2023). Still, I claim that cross-national comparison illustrates a meaningful cross-national tendency, which is useful under the assumption that such sampling bias is not systematically uneven across countries. Seemingly constant tendencies over the target period manifested in Fig. 3.4 suggest the gaps represent systematic patterns beyond the reflection of short-term factors such as anxiety about the infection risk. One may also suspect selection bias in recruiting survey participants via Facebook, such as the urban–rural or ethnic divides that hinder certain categories of people from participating in the survey. This, however, should work as the overrepresentation of urban and non-indigenous populations in the sample and hence tend to overestimate test capacity in the given country. Overestimation is likelier in countries like Bolivia, Ecuador, Guatemala, and Peru for relatively higher indigenous population shares and Honduras, Nicaragua, and Paraguay for relatively lower urbanization rates. Since these are ranked higher in the *non-tested ratios* and *percentages*, I assume my findings based on the relative ranking remain unchanged. One exception might be Paraguay, which scores low in the two indicators of test capacity limitations, which I suspect is due to the small total sample size (n = 466), the second smallest among all the countries, and the possible overrepresentation of urban residents.

This study discloses a clear alignment between lower non-tested percentages and lower CFRs. Still, the mechanism that links test capacity limitations with CFR is unclear. Test capacity improvement may resonate with strong health infrastructure or at least reliable health policy design and implementation facing an unprecedented crisis. These may be distinctive from state capacity in general and possibly specific to the health sector. Measuring legibility is a challenge, especially in a critical moment like the pandemic when states all over the world are pressured to not only collect information but also rescue people suffering from severe symptoms. Political maneuvers can further undermine the reliability of officially reported data. However, state preparedness can be a defining factor in eventually saving the lives of people. Recounting the limitation in this specific aspect of state capacity must pave the road for necessary reforms in the post-pandemic era.

Acknowledgments The analysis of this chapter was made possible thanks to the University of Maryland, in collaboration with Meta Platforms, Inc., who generously shared the daily survey data. I also appreciate productive comments on an earlier manuscript by participants in a panel at the IPSA Conference in July 2023, a workshop in Colegio de Mexico in March 2024, and a workshop at Waseda University in September 2024. This study was supported by JSPS KAKENHI Grant No. 20KK0024 and No. 23K17283.

Supplementary Files

S3.1 Sample size for each country in the CTIS data: June 27–December 27, 2020

Argentina	3453	Dominican Republic	941	Nicaragua	229
Bolivia	1437	Ecuador	2685	Panama	516
Brazil	22,857	El Salvador	625	Paraguay	466
Chile	2309	Guatemala	849	Peru	3611
Colombia	3823	Honduras	929	Uruguay	544
Costa Rica	603	Mexico	13,989	Venezuela	1040

Source: Author

S3.2 Time-series sample size fluctuation in the CTIS data. Source: Author based on the CTIS data

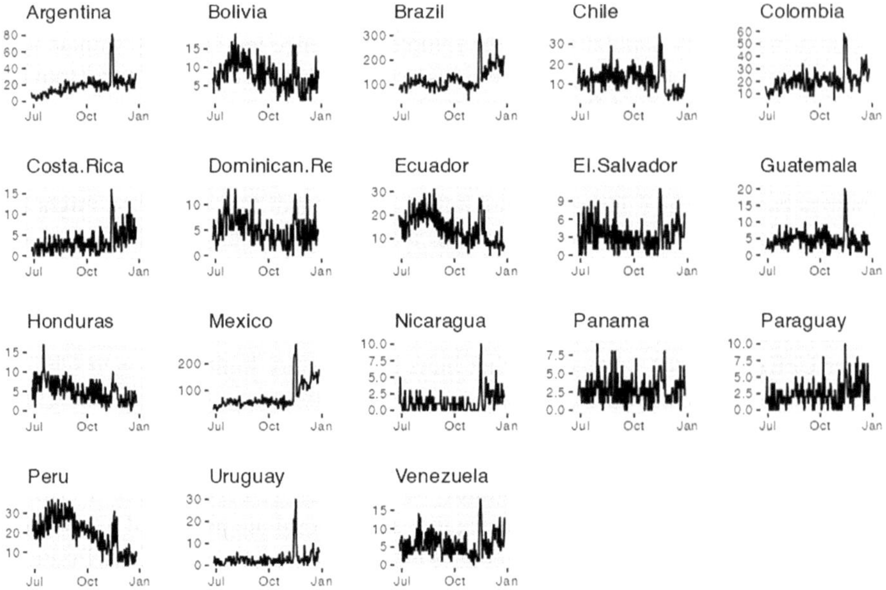

S3.3 Oxford stringency index. Dashed lines indicate the target period of this chapter. The index is a composite of nine metrics: school closures; workplace closures; cancellation of public events; restrictions on public gatherings; closures of public transport; stay-at-home requirements; public information campaigns; restrictions on internal movements; and international travel controls. Source: Hale et al. (2021); The data was retrieved from https://ourworldindata.org/covid-stringency-index (last access, June 30, 2023)

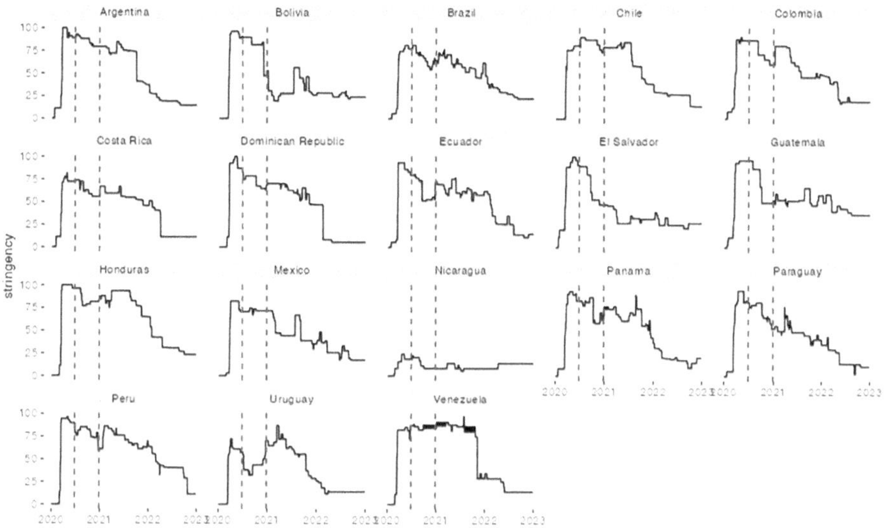

S3.4 Test policies. Dashed lines indicate the target period of this chapter. 0 = No policy. 1 = Only those who both (a) have symptoms AND (b) meet specific criteria (e.g., key workers, admitted to hospital, came into contact with a known case, returned from overseas). 2 = Testing of anyone showing COVID-19 symptoms. 3 = Open public testing (e.g., "drive through" testing available to asymptomatic people). Source: Hale et al. (2021); The data was retrieved from https://ourworldindata.org/covid-testing-contact-tracing (last access, June 18, 2023)

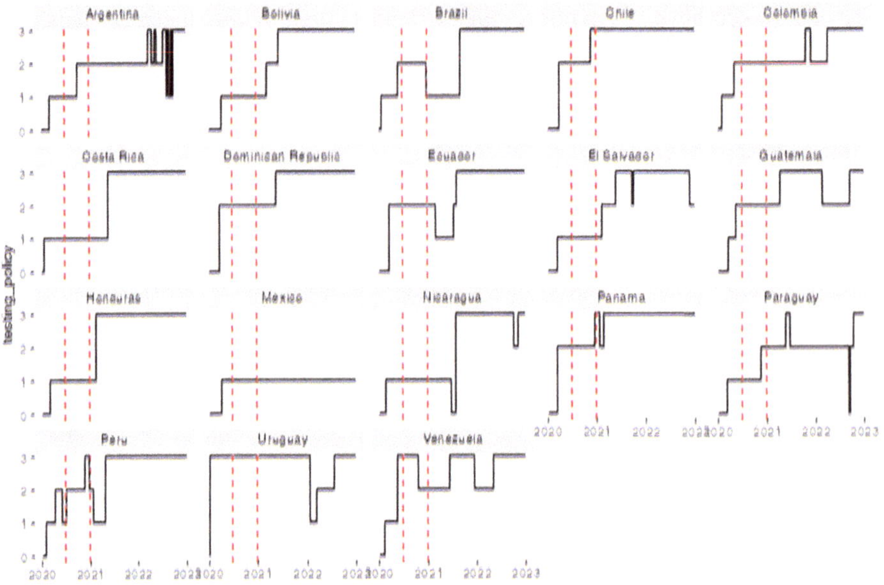

S3.5 Contact tracing policy. Dashed lines indicate the target period of this chapter. 0 = No contact tracing. 1 = Limited contact tracing—not done for all cases. 2 = Comprehensive contact tracing—done for all cases. Source: Hale et al. (2021); The data was retrieved from https://ourworldindata.org/covid-testing-contact-tracing (last access, June 18, 2023)

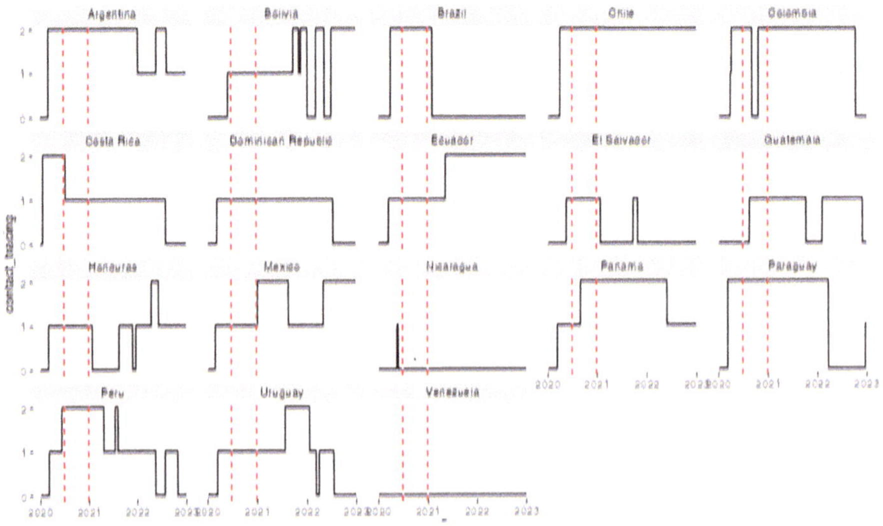

S3.6 Comparing non-tested percentage and ratio. Source: Author

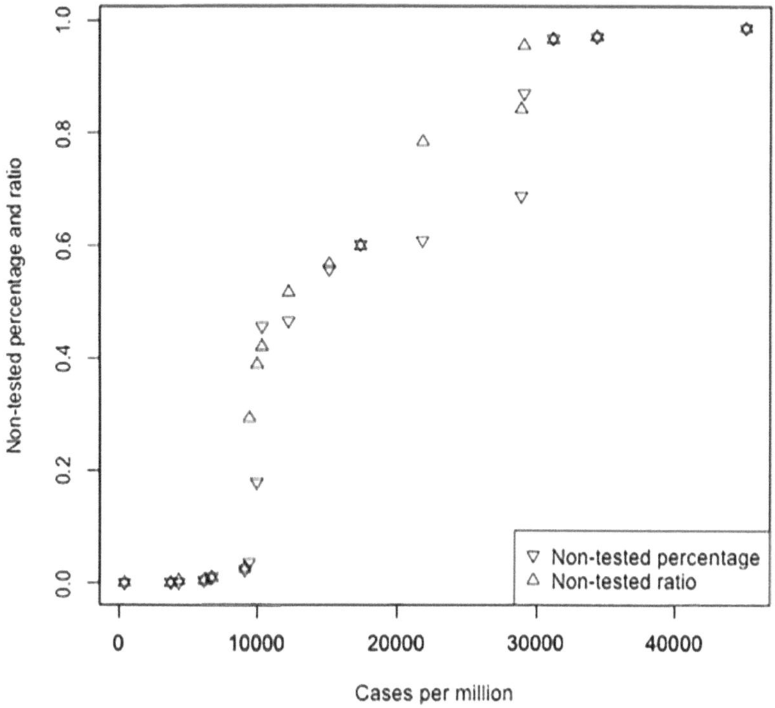

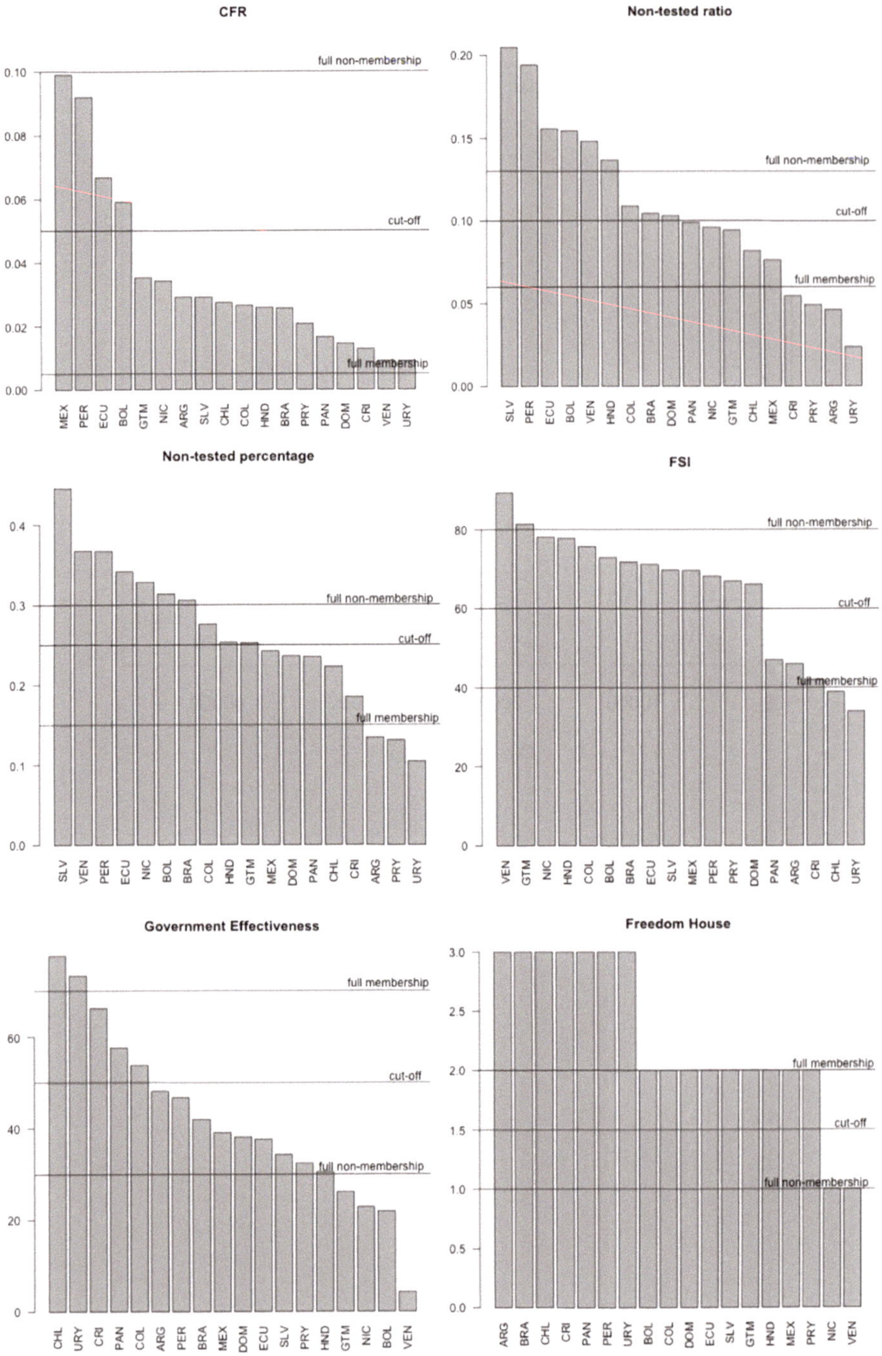

S3.7 Outcome and conditions with assigned values for calibration. Source: Author

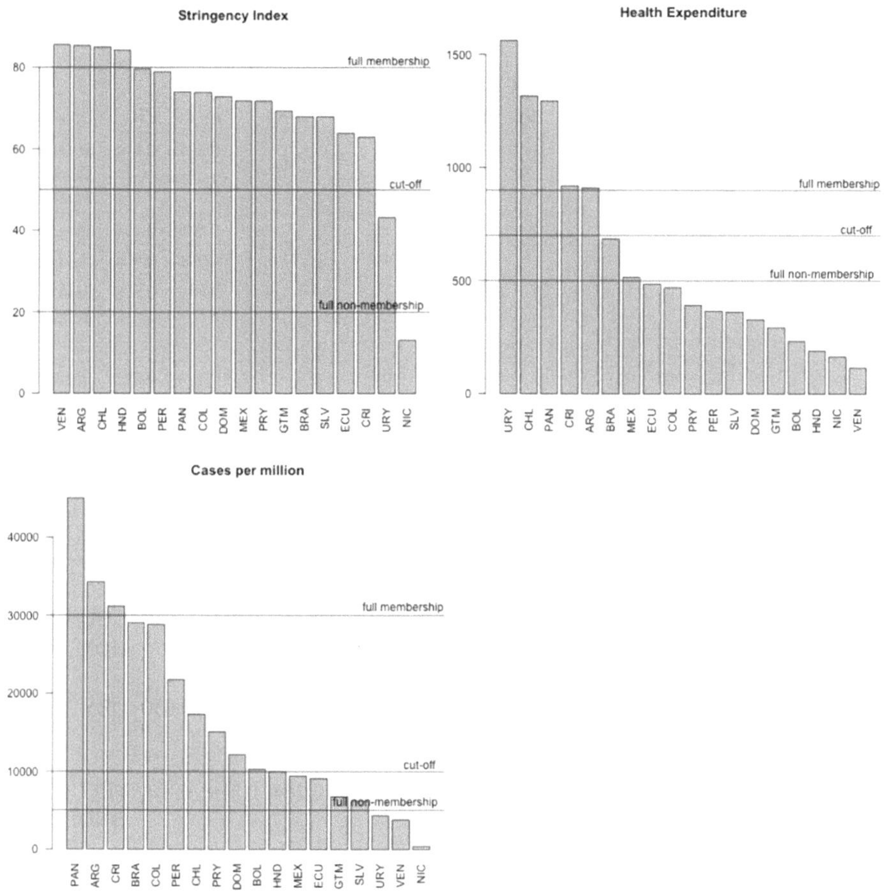

S3.8 Truth table

Non-tested percentage	Non-tested ratio	FH	FSI	Stringency	Gov Eff	Health expenditure	Cases	Outcome (CFR)	incl	PRI	Cases
0	1	0	0	0	0	0	0	1	1.000	1.000	Nicaragua
1	1	1	1	1	1	1	1	1	0.997	0.995	Chile, Costa Rica, Panama
1	1	1	1	1	0	1	1	1	0.992	0.983	Argentina
1	1	1	1	0	1	1	0	1	0.990	0.985	Uruguay
0	0	0	0	1	0	0	0	1	0.990	0.984	Venezuela
1	0	1	0	1	0	0	1	1	0.941	0.889	Dominican Republic

(continued)

Non-tested percentage	Non-tested ratio	FH	FSI	Stringency	Gov Eff	Health expenditure	Cases	Outcome (CFR)	incl	PRI	Cases
0	0	1	0	1	0	0	0	1	0.827	0.674	Ecuador, El Salvador, Honduras
1	1	1	0	1	0	0	1	1	0.816	0.708	Paraguay
0	0	1	0	1	1	0	1	0	0.796	0.594	Colombia
0	0	1	0	1	0	0	1	0	0.767	0.578	Bolivia, Brazil,Peru
0	1	1	0	1	0	0	0	0	0.764	0.593	Guatemala
1	1	1	0	1	0	0	0	0	0.744	0.586	Mexico

Source: Author

S3.9 Test for sufficiency: complex solutions

	inclS	PRI	covS	covU	Cases
non-tested percentage * non-tested ratio * FH * FSI * Stringency * Health expenditure * Cases	0.967	0.957	0.235	0.211	ARG, CHL, COL, PAN
non-tested percentage * FH * ~FSI * Stringency * ~GovEff * ~Health expenditure * Cases	0.859	0.784	0.177	0.076	DOM, PRY
non-tested percentage * non-tested ratio * FH * FSI * ~Stringency * GovEff * Health expenditure * ~Cases	0.990	0.985	0.072	0.050	URY
~non-tested percentage * ~non-tested ratio * ~FSI * Stringency * ~GovEff * ~Health expenditure * ~Cases	0.854	0.764	0.319	0.218	ECU, SAL, HND, VEN

Source: Author
* logical multiplication, ~ the condition's absence

References

Adcock, R., & Collier, D. (2001). Measurement validity: A shared standard for qualitative and quantitative research. *The American Political Science Review, 95*(3), 529–546.

Alfano, V., & Ercolano, S. (2022). Stay at home! Governance quality and effectiveness of lockdown. *Social Indicators Research, 159*(1), 101–123. https://doi.org/10.1007/s11205-021-02742-3

Alicea-Planas, J., Trudeau, J. M., & Vásquez Mazariegos, W. F. (2021). COVID-19 risk perceptions and social distancing practice in Latin America. *Hispanic Health Care International, 19*(4), 254–259. https://doi.org/10.1177/1540415320985141

An, B. Y., & Tang, S.-Y. (2020). Lessons from COVID-19 responses in East Asia: Institutional infrastructure and enduring policy instruments. *The American Review of Public Administration, 50*(6–7), 790–800. https://doi.org/10.1177/0275074020943707

Aruguete, N., Calvo, E., Cantú, F., Ley, S., Scartascini, C., & Ventura, T. (2021). Partisan cues and perceived risks: The effect of partisan social media frames during the COVID-19 crisis in Mexico. *Journal of Elections, Public Opinion and Parties, 31*(Suppl 1), 82–95. https://doi.org/10.1080/17457289.2021.1924740

Baumgartner, M. (2015). Parsimony and causality. *Quality & Quantity, 49*(2), 839–856. https://doi.org/10.1007/s11135-014-0026-7

Benítez, M. A., Velasco, C., Sequeira, A. R., Henríquez, J., Menezes, F. M., & Paolucci, F. (2020). Responses to COVID-19 in five Latin American countries. *Health Policy and Technology, 9*(4), 525–559. https://doi.org/10.1016/j.hlpt.2020.08.014

Bidegain, G., Freigedo, M., & Fuentes, G. (2021). The Uruguayan State's structure and the management of the pandemic. In M. Fernandez & C. Machado (Eds.), *COVID-19's political challenges in Latin America* (pp. 67–84). Springer International. https://doi.org/10.1007/978-3-030-77602-2_6

Bosancianu, C. M., Hilbig, H., Humphreys, M., Kc, S., Lieber, N., & Scacco, A. (2020). *Political and social correlates of Covid-19 mortality* [Preprint]. SocArXiv. https://doi.org/10.31235/osf.io/ub3zd

Brambor, T., Goenaga, A., Lindvall, J., & Teorell, J. (2020). The lay of the land: Information capacity and the modern state. *Comparative Political Studies, 53*(2), 175–213. https://doi.org/10.1177/0010414019843432

Brinks, D. M., Levitsky, S., & Murillo, M. V. (Eds.). (2020). *The politics of institutional weakness in Latin America*. Cambridge University Press. https://doi.org/10.1017/9781108776608

Calvo, E., & Ventura, T. (2021). Will I get COVID-19? Partisanship, social media frames, and perceptions of health risk in Brazil. *Latin American Politics and Society, 63*(1), 1–26. https://doi.org/10.1017/lap.2020.30

Capano, G. (2020). Policy design and state capacity in the COVID-19 emergency in Italy: If you are not prepared for the (un)expected, you can be only what you already are. *Policy and Society, 39*(3), 326–344. https://doi.org/10.1080/14494035.2020.1783790

Capano, G., Howlett, M., Jarvis, D. S. L., Ramesh, M., & Goyal, N. (2020). Mobilizing policy (in) capacity to fight COVID-19: Understanding variations in state responses. *Policy and Society, 39*(3), 285–308. https://doi.org/10.1080/14494035.2020.1787628

Castorena, O., Lupu, N., Schade, M., & Zechmeister, E. J. (2023). Online surveys in Latin America. *PS: Political Science & Politics, 56*(2), 273–280. https://doi.org/10.1017/S1049096522001287

CEPAL. (2020, May). *Las restricciones a la exportación de productos médicos dificultan los esfuerzos por contener la enfermedad por coronavirus (COVID-19) en América Latina y el Caribe*. https://www.cepal.org/es/publicaciones/45510-restricciones-la-exportacion-productos-medicos-dificultan-esfuerzos-contener-la

Cheng, M. P., Papenburg, J., Desjardins, M., Kanjilal, S., Quach, C., Libman, M., Dittrich, S., & Yansouni, C. P. (2020). Diagnostic testing for severe acute respiratory syndrome–related coronavirus 2: A narrative review. *Annals of Internal Medicine, 172*(11), 726–734. https://doi.org/10.7326/M20-1301

Cyr, J., Bianchi, M., González, L., & Perini, A. (2021). Governing a pandemic: Assessing the role of collaboration on Latin American responses to the COVID-19 Crisis. *Journal of Politics in Latin America, 13*(3), 290–327. https://doi.org/10.1177/1866802X211049250

Delgado-Diaz, D. J., Zuniga-Gutierrez, M. A., Narh, C. A., & Richards, J. S. (2021). *Opinion: Early COVID-19 testing in Peru and its implications on transmission* [Preprint]. Open Science Framework. https://doi.org/10.31219/osf.io/nkc25

Farge, E., & Revill, J. (2020, March 17). "Test, test, test": WHO chief's coronavirus message to world. *Reuters*. https://www.reuters.com/article/us-healthcare-coronavirus-who-idUSKBN2132S4

Gisselquist, R. M., & Vaccaro, A. (2023). COVID-19 and the state: Exploring a puzzling relationship in the early stages of the pandemic. *Journal of International Development, 35*(5), 800–819. https://doi.org/10.1002/jid.3702

González-Bustamante, B. (2021). Evolution and early government responses to COVID-19 in South America. *World Development, 137*, 105180. https://doi.org/10.1016/j.worlddev.2020.105180

Gramacho, W. G., & Turgeon, M. (2021). When politics collides with public health: COVID-19 vaccine country of origin and vaccination acceptance in Brazil. *Vaccine, 39*(19), 2608–2612. https://doi.org/10.1016/j.vaccine.2021.03.080

Hale, T., Angrist, N., Goldszmidt, R., Kira, B., Petherick, A., Phillips, T., Webster, S., Cameron-Blake, E., Hallas, L., Majumdar, S., & Tatlow, H. (2021). A global panel database of pandemic policies (Oxford COVID-19 Government Response Tracker). *Nature Human Behaviour, 5*(4), 529–538. https://doi.org/10.1038/s41562-021-01079-8

Hasell, J., Mathieu, E., Beltekian, D., Macdonald, B., Giattino, C., Ortiz-Ospina, E., Roser, M., & Ritchie, H. (2020). A cross-country database of COVID-19 testing. *Scientific Data, 7*(1), 345. https://doi.org/10.1038/s41597-020-00688-8

Jarquin, M., & Marti i Puig, S. (2021). Nicaragua: Denying the health crisis and the political crisis. In M. Fernandez & C. Machado (Eds.), *COVID-19's Political challenges in Latin America* (pp. 35–45). Springer International.

Kameda, K., Barbeitas, M. M., Caetano, R., Löwy, I., Oliveira, A. C. D. D., Corrêa, M. C. D. V., & Cassier, M. (2021). Testing COVID-19 in Brazil: Fragmented efforts and challenges to expand diagnostic capacity at the Brazilian Unified National Health System. *Cadernos de Saúde Pública, 37*(3), e00277420. https://doi.org/10.1590/0102-311x00277420

Kurtz, M. J. (2013). *Latin American state building in comparative perspective: Social foundations of institutional order*. Cambridge University Press.

Lee, M. M., & Zhang, N. (2017). Legibility and the informational foundations of state capacity. *The Journal of Politics, 79*(1), 118–132. https://doi.org/10.1086/688053

Luna, J. P., & Soifer, H. D. (2017). Capturing sub-national variation in state capacity: A survey-based approach. *American Behavioral Scientist, 61*(8), 887–907. https://doi.org/10.1177/0002764217720964

Mahoney, J. (2010). *Colonialism and development: Spanish America in comparative perspective*. Cambridge University Press. https://doi.org/10.1017/CBO9780511750328

Medeiros, A., Bertholini, F., & Pereira, C. (2021). Identity versus fear of death: Political polarization under the COVID-19 pandemic in Brazil. In M. Fernandez & C. Machado (Eds.), *COVID-19's political challenges in Latin America* (pp. 133–145). Springer International. https://doi.org/10.1007/978-3-030-77602-2_10

Mercer, T. R., & Salit, M. (2021). Testing at scale during the COVID-19 pandemic. *Nature Reviews Genetics, 22*(7), 415–426. https://doi.org/10.1038/s41576-021-00360-w

Paniz-Mondolfi, A. E., Sordillo, E. M., Márquez-Colmenarez, M. C., Delgado-Noguera, L. A., & Rodriguez-Morales, A. J. (2020). The arrival of SARS-CoV-2 in Venezuela. *The Lancet, 395*(10236), e85–e86. https://doi.org/10.1016/S0140-6736(20)31053-9

Pearson, A. A., Prado, A. M., & Colburn, F. D. (2021). The puzzle of COVID-19 in Central America and Panama. *Journal of Global Health, 11*, 03077. https://doi.org/10.7189/jogh.11.03077

Peeling, R. W., Olliaro, P. L., Boeras, D. I., & Fongwen, N. (2021). Scaling up COVID-19 rapid antigen tests: Promises and challenges. *The Lancet Infectious Diseases, 21*(9), e290–e295. https://doi.org/10.1016/S1473-3099(21)00048-7

Piazza, K. S., & Schwier, A. (2021). Ready, set, vaccine: The path to COVID-19 recovery in Latin America. *Revista Latinoamericana de Opinión Pública, 10*(2), 179–190. https://doi.org/10.14201/rlop.26940

Pollán, M., Pérez-Gómez, B., Pastor-Barriuso, R., Oteo, J., Hernán, M. A., Pérez-Olmeda, M., Sanmartín, J. L., Fernández-García, A., Cruz, I., Fernández De Larrea, N., Molina, M., Rodríguez-Cabrera, F., Martín, M., Merino-Amador, P., León Paniagua, J., Muñoz-Montalvo, J. F., Blanco, F., Yotti, R., Blanco, F., et al. (2020). Prevalence of SARS-CoV-2 in Spain (ENE-COVID): A nationwide, population-based seroepidemiological study. *The Lancet, 396*(10250), 535–544. https://doi.org/10.1016/S0140-6736(20)31483-5

Ragin, C. C. (2008). *Redesigning social inquiry: Fuzzy sets and beyond*. University of Chicago Press.

Rannan-Eliya, R. P., Wijemunige, N., Gunawardana, J. R. N. A., Amarasinghe, S. N., Sivagnanam, I., Fonseka, S., Kapuge, Y., & Sigera, C. P. (2021). Increased intensity of PCR testing reduced

COVID-19 transmission within countries during the first pandemic wave: Study examines increased intensity of reverse transcription–polymerase chain reaction (PCR) testing and its impact on COVID-19 transmission. *Health Affairs, 40*(1), 70–81. https://doi.org/10.1377/hlthaff.2020.01409

Saylor, R. (2014). *State building in boom times: Commodities and coalitions in Latin America and Africa*. Oxford University Press.

Schaefer, B. M., Resende, R. C., Epitácio, S. S. F., & Aleixo, M. T. (2020). Government actions against the new coronavirus: Evidence from the Brazilian states. *Revista de Administração Pública, 54*(5), 1429–1445. https://doi.org/10.1590/0034-761220200503x

Schneider, C. Q., & Wagemann, C. (2012). *Set-theoretic methods for the social sciences: A guide to qualitative comparative analysis*. Cambridge University Press.

Scohy, A., Anantharajah, A., Bodéus, M., Kabamba-Mukadi, B., Verroken, A., & Rodriguez-Villalobos, H. (2020). Low performance of rapid antigen detection test as frontline testing for COVID-19 diagnosis. *Journal of Clinical Virology, 129*, 104455. https://doi.org/10.1016/j.jcv.2020.104455

Scott, J. C. (2008). *Seeing like a state: How certain schemes to improve the human condition have failed*. Yale University Press.

Serikbayeva, B., Abdulla, K., & Oskenbayev, Y. (2021). State capacity in responding to COVID-19. *International Journal of Public Administration, 44*(11–12), 920–930. https://doi.org/10.1080/01900692.2020.1850778

Soifer, H. D. (2015). *State building in Latin America*. Cambridge University Press. http://ezproxy.library.qmul.ac.uk/login?url=https://doi.org/10.1017/CBO9781316257289

Taylor, L. (2020). Uruguay is winning against covid-19. This is how. *BMJ*, m3575. https://doi.org/10.1136/bmj.m3575

Trudeau, J. M., Alicea-Planas, J., & Vásquez, W. F. (2020). The value of COVID-19 tests in Latin America. *Economics & Human Biology, 39*, 100931. https://doi.org/10.1016/j.ehb.2020.100931

Urrunaga-Pastor, D., Bendezu-Quispe, G., Herrera-Añazco, P., Uyen-Cateriano, A., Toro-Huamanchumo, C. J., Rodriguez-Morales, A. J., Hernandez, A. V., & Benites-Zapata, V. A. (2021). Cross-sectional analysis of COVID-19 vaccine intention, perceptions and hesitancy across Latin America and the Caribbean. *Travel Medicine and Infectious Disease, 41*, 102059. https://doi.org/10.1016/j.tmaid.2021.102059

Yashar, D. J. (2018). *Homicidal ecologies: Illicit economies and complicit states in Latin America*. Cambridge University Press.

Chapter 4
Assessing the Impact of Central Government Announcements on Mask-Wearing Compliance in Latin America During COVID-19

Takahiro Miyachi

4.1 Introduction

The use of masks as a non-pharmaceutical intervention to reduce the spread of COVID-19 has become a common practice worldwide since the onset of the pandemic in 2020. Masks have gained significant acceptance due to their affordability and their ability to allow people who may face challenges in maintaining home isolation to go outside while still reducing the risk of infection. Although there is some debate about their precise preventive effectiveness, numerous studies have acknowledged their role in lowering infection risk (Brüssow & Zuber, 2022; Boulos et al., 2023).

A wide range of research has examined the factors influencing mask-wearing behavior at both individual and societal levels. Previous studies have highlighted the impact of personal characteristics, such as gender (Haischer et al., 2020), race (Papageorge et al., 2021; Heame & Niño, 2021), age (Capraro & Barcelo, 2020; Palmer & Peterson, 2020), education level (Palmer & Peterson, 2020; Rieger, 2020), political ideology (Palmer & Peterson, 2020; Pew Research Center, 2020), residential area (Palmer & Peterson, 2020; Pew Research Center, 2020; Callaghan et al., 2021), and health consciousness (Callaghan et al., 2021; He et al., 2021). Additionally, research has identified social conformity pressure as a factor wherein individuals are influenced to wear or not wear masks based on the prevailing behavior in their surroundings (Rieger, 2020; Sakakibara & Ozono, 2021; Yang et al., 2022).

Despite the extensive body of research, the specific influence of government announcements on mask-wearing compliance remains insufficiently explored.

T. Miyachi (✉)
The University of Tokyo, Tokyo, Japan
e-mail: miyachi@anthro.c.u-tokyo.ac.jp

I. Okada (ed.), *COVID-19 and State Capacity in Latin America*, Latin American Societies, https://doi.org/10.1007/978-3-032-15572-6_4

Haischer et al. (2020) highlight the significant role of government communications through a survey in 14 commercial centers across Massachusetts, United States, suggesting the potential impact of public announcements. However, it is unclear whether this effect extends to broader contexts. Yang et al. (2022) employ a game-theory model that incorporates policy stringency, social conformity (categorized as loose or tight), and COVID-19 case data as determinants of mask-wearing ratios. By analyzing data from 26 countries across different regions between February 2020 and October 2021, the study concludes that countries with loose social conformity tend to respond more rapidly to policy changes, while those with tight social conformity exhibit delayed reactions—policy stringency only becomes effective after a certain threshold of mask-wearing is achieved, and reductions in stringency result in gradual declines in compliance. While the study identifies a general trend in policy effects, it does not investigate the nuanced dynamics of individual policy implementations.

This chapter aims to reassess the importance of government decisions regarding mask-wearing. When a government recommends mask usage, the reasons behind an individual's decision to wear a mask can vary. A person might wear a mask to comply with government directives, or they might choose to wear one due to inadequate public healthcare services, which could indicate a lack of state capacity. Moreover, in cases where the government strongly advocates for mask-wearing during a rapid spread of infection, it can be challenging to distinguish whether the increase in mask-wearing is driven by trust in the government or by individuals' voluntary, self-protective responses to the escalating contagion.

It is also important to recognize that changes in mask-wearing rates can result from multiple underlying causes. Attributing these changes solely to government decisions would be an oversimplification. Equifinality, which acknowledges that different factors can interact and contribute to the outcome of increased mask-wearing rates, is likely at play.

To contextualize the effect of state capacity, Latin America provides an ideal region for study. While the 20 countries in the region share similar Latin cultural backgrounds and historical processes, such as the timing of independence and economic stagnation in the nineteenth century and the decade of 1980s, they differ in key political characteristics, including the endurance of democratic regimes and, as discussed later, state capacity. Indeed, political science has often viewed Latin America as a valuable field for comparative research. This chapter also appraises this quality and selects Latin American countries as the object of analysis.

Mask-wearing announcements may have both short-term and long-term effects. This chapter focuses on the short-term effects, which are more likely to be accurately captured compared to long-term effects, where controlling for potential covariates is challenging. To address the research question of this chapter, two steps are necessary. The first step involves quantifying the changes in mask-wearing that occur in response to government policy changes. The second step entails identifying the factors that determine the magnitude of these changes.

4.2 Step One: Quantifying Changes in Mask-Wearing

To capture shifts in individuals' mask-wearing behavior, this study relies on data from the University of Maryland Social Data Science Center Global COVID-19 Trends and Impact Survey (CTIS). The CTIS administers online surveys on COVID-19 using Facebook as a platform across multiple countries globally, collecting over 100 million responses from April 2020 to 2022. The start and end dates of data collection vary by country. From this dataset, responses meeting the following two criteria are extracted:

1. The response is from a Latin American country, as indicated by the "country_agg" column in CTIS.
2. The response period spans 10 days before and after the starting point (SP), which is defined as 3 days after the policy change date at 12:00 PM. For instance, if a policy change occurs on October 10th, the SP would be October 13th at 12:00 PM. Thus, responses from October 3rd, 12:00 PM to October 23rd, 11:59 AM are included. Policy change dates are identified using The Oxford COVID-19 Government Response Tracker (OxCGRT) (Hale et al., 2021). The rationale for setting the SP after the policy change date will be explained later.

Tables 4.1 and 4.2 present the policy changes of interest for analysis, along with the corresponding number of responses. These policy changes are categorized into

Table 4.1 Extracted responses from CTIS: Encouraging announcement

No.	Country	SP Date	*N*	No.	Country	SP Date	*N*
1	Bolivia	20/5/4	24,809	20	Honduras	21/12/23	3321
2	Bolivia	20/6/3	33,870	21	Haiti	20/5/26	2064
3	Bolivia	20/12/11	12,185	22	Mexico	22/1/13	135,733
4	Chile	20/12/11	28,158	23	Mexico	22/6/10	51,363
5	Chile	21/4/29	24,336	24	Nicaragua	21/2/19	3999
6	Colombia	21/4/8	45,945	25	Nicaragua	21/6/17	2969
7	Colombia	21/10/21	23,050	26	Nicaragua	21/10/4	5442
8	Costa Rica	20/6/25	23,874	27	Panama	20/6/5	9625
9	Costa Rica	20/11/5	5005	28	Peru	20/8/4	37,857
10	Dom. Rep	20/5/4	12,717	29	Peru	21/2/26	29,275
11	Dom. Rep	21/5/24	6573	30	Peru	21/12/9	11,706
12	Dom. Rep	22/3/10	2213	31	Paraguay	20/7/31	8518
13	Ecuador	21/6/29	11,871	32	Paraguay	20/11/30	6054
14	Guatemala	21/5/3	7792	33	Paraguay	21/6/18	4316
15	Guatemala	21/7/16	9096	34	El Salvador	21/10/28	8638
16	Guatemala	22/2/5	6551	35	Uruguay	20/5/31	18,511
17	Guatemala	22/3/19	5084	36	Uruguay	22/4/3	4497
18	Honduras	21/5/7	5155	37	Venezuela	20/11/3	6976
19	Honduras	20/5/24	18,727	38	Venezuela	22/1/7	10,526

The SP Date follows the format yy/mm/dd. Dom. Rep: Dominican Republic.

Table 4.2 Extracted responses from CTIS: Discouraging announcement

No.	Country	SP Date	*N*	No.	Country	SP Date	*N*
1	Argentina	22/5/13	21,542	20	Mexico	22/2/24	65,858
2	Brazil	21/9/3	158,931	21	Mexico	22/5/5	48,919
3	Brazil	22/3/22	99,433	22	Nicaragua	21/3/26	3855
4	Chile	20/12/18	29,056	23	Nicaragua	21/5/27	3971
5	Chile	22/4/17	11,961	24	Nicaragua	21/9/4	7154
6	Colombia	20/9/4	43,881	25	Nicaragua	21/10/21	4089
7	Colombia	22/3/4	17,107	26	Nicaragua	22/4/13	1007
8	Costa Rica	22/4/4	4174	27	Panama	22/3/31	1637
9	Dom. Rep.	21/9/28	3271	28	Paraguay	20/11/17	3590
10	Dom. Rep.	22/2/19	2528	29	Paraguay	21/6/11	5233
11	Dom. Rep.	22/3/24	2187	30	Paraguay	22/1/26	3390
12	Dom. Rep.	22/4/12	1210	31	Paraguay	22/5/20	1536
13	Ecuador	21/5/29	16,347	32	Peru	20/10/4	18,801
14	Guatemala	21/7/9	9560	33	Peru	21/11/27	12,591
15	Guatemala	21/11/12	6004	34	Peru	22/5/4	9060
16	Guatemala	21/12/10	4997	35	Uruguay	22/3/11	4762
17	Honduras	21/6/25	3452	36	Uruguay	22/4/22	4154
18	Honduras	21/11/30	2904	37	Venezuela	21/12/1	10,070
19	Mexico	21/12/2	77,501				

The SP Date follows the format yy/mm/dd. Dom. Rep: Dominican Republic.

those that encourage mask-wearing and those that discourage it. During the periods covered by CTIS, there were 38 confirmed policy changes in the former category and 37 in the latter.

The dependent variable in this analysis is the response to questions regarding mask-wearing. In question C5 of the CTIS survey, participants were asked about the frequency of mask-wearing during the past 7 days, with six response options ranging from "never wear a mask" (option 1) to "always wear a mask" (option 5). Option 6 is "always stay at home." If a government announcement is effective, a change in mask-wearing behavior would appear by the fourth day after the announcement date. This is why SP is set 3 days after the policy change date.

A conventional approach to identifying factors that increase the likelihood of selecting different response options, such as those regarding mask-wearing, is multinomial logistic regression analysis. However, this method assumes a consistent trend before and after an intervention. Recent social science studies have addressed this limitation by incorporating experimental designs. This paper introduces the regression discontinuity design (RDD) to detect the gap in mask-wearing frequency at SP between the pre-SP trend and the post-SP trend.

The RDD is traditionally applied to analyses with continuous dependent variables. Since the dependent variable in this study is categorical, using the conventional RDD would require assuming that the categorical options are continuous values. However, the option "always stay at home" does not align with the other five options. While it might seem logical to place "always stay at home" at the highest level of protection, the best approach is to treat all these options as categorical. To address this, this study uses the categorical RDD developed by Xu (2017). The local average treatment effect (LATE) measured by the categorical RDD represents the percentage change of choosing the target option. As widely known, using fine-grained categories as a dependent variable in logit analysis can lead to inaccurate results by reducing the number of cases in each category. To avoid this problem, this paper employs a three-stage multinomial logit model, where options 1 to 3 are categorized as "non-wearing," options 4 and 5 as "wearing," and option 6 as "staying at home."

The explanatory variable of interest, also called the running variable in the RDD, is the time variable. It measures the time distance between SP and the date of the answer. As the data analyzed here cover 10 days before and after the SP, the value of time ranges from −10 to 10. The LATE represents the difference in the probability of "wearing" at a *time* value of 0. This paper will have a total of 75 LATEs, with 38 from the mask-encouraging announcement cases and 37 from the mask-discouraging cases.

It is noteworthy that Xu (2017) does not control for other covariates beyond the running variable because it "is not necessary for identification of the causal effect" (Xu, 2017, p. 11). Imbens and Lemieux (2008, pp. 625–626), whom Xu (2017) cites in support of this argument, state that "the variance reduction will be relatively small unless the contribution to the adjusted R^2 from the additional regressors is substantial." This paper replicates Miyachi (2023), which employed a multinomial logit analysis with the aforementioned three-category dependent variables, to identify covariates that improve adjusted R^2 by more than 0.1, the threshold set by Cohen (1989, pp. 413–414) for medium improvement. The results indicate that there are no such variables in the 75 cases.

Figures 4.1 and 4.2 illustrate the error bars representing the 95% confidence intervals for the LATEs across the 75 cases analyzed. Each case is denoted by an abbreviation corresponding to the country and the specific period covered. For instance, the case for Bolivia from April 4 to April 24, 2020, is labeled as "Bol200404_200424". Out of the 38 cases involving a policy shift toward encouraging mask usage, 7 cases demonstrated statistically significant positive LATEs, while 1 case indicated a negative LATE. Conversely, in the 37 cases where policies reduced the encouragement of mask-wearing, only 2 cases, both originating from Brazil, exhibited negative LATEs. By contrast, interestingly, 6 cases showed positive LATEs. Overall, announcements promoting mask-wearing are more effective in eliciting the desired behavior change than those discouraging mask usage, which largely failed to significantly alter public behavior regarding mask-wearing.

4.3 Step Two: Identification of the Conditions

The second step of this inquiry focuses on identifying the factors that influence the coefficients determined in the first step. As mentioned earlier, it is essential to recognize that the significance and magnitude of these coefficients may vary based on

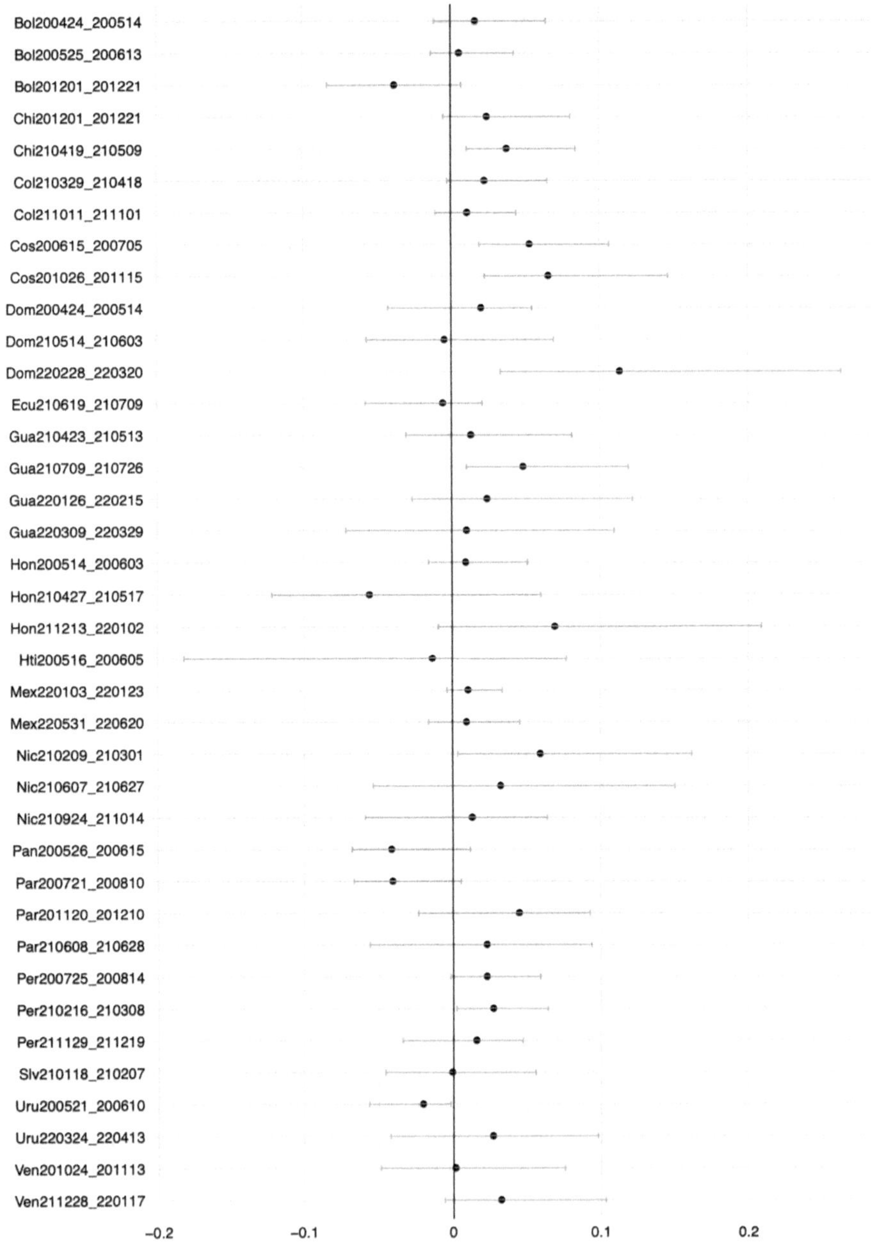

Fig. 4.1 LATEs of the encouraging announcements ($n = 38$)

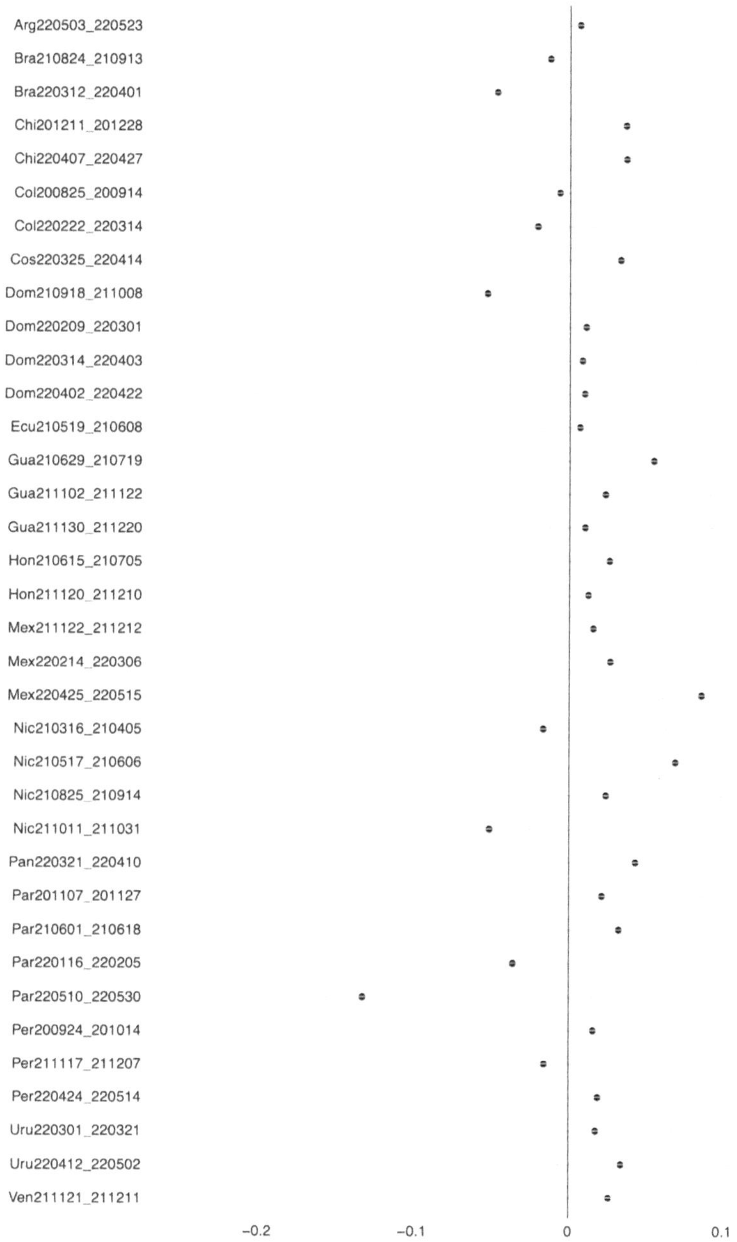

Fig. 4.2 LATEs of the discouraging announcements ($n = 37$)

different factors in each case. To address this issue of result consistency, using fuzzy-set qualitative comparative analysis (fsQCA) is beneficial. Since Step One found that the government's discouraging mask-wearing announcements were ineffective, the analysis will focus on the cases involving encouraging announcements.

4.3.1 Outcome and Conditions

The outcome is the LATE obtained in Step One. Cases that do not meet the 5% significance level are assigned a coefficient value of 0, while the remaining cases retain their respective coefficient values. For determining the number of independent variables, this study follows best practices in QCA, which recommend setting it as the smallest power of 2 that exceeds the number of cases (Rihoux & Ragin, 2008). As explained later, the number of cases is 29, which is 9 fewer than 38 due to the lack of data for a particular condition. Consequently, the number of variables should be limited to five or fewer. The following five factors are considered as conditions:

Government Effectiveness (*ge*) State capacity has attracted scholarly attention in analyzing public policies related to COVID-19. While governments worldwide have pledged to tackle the pandemic, the credibility of these commitments varies across countries. The World Governance Indicators (WGI) of the World Bank, one of the most frequently cited indexes of state capacity for political analysis, includes "government effectiveness" as one of its components. It "captures perceptions of the quality of public services, the quality of the civil service and the degree of its independence from political pressures, the quality of policy formulation and implementation, and the credibility of the government's commitment to such policies" (World Bank, 2023). Although its subcomponents include aspects not directly related to COVID-19, such as satisfaction with public transportation services, it serves as the best proxy for state capacity. The value theoretically ranges from −2.5 to 2.5, with 0 representing a standard level of effectiveness among the country-year-based samples. For reference, as of the 2022 data, the highest value is 2.14 for Singapore, and the lowest is −2.39 for South Sudan. Among Latin American countries in the same year, the highest is 0.85 for Uruguay, and the lowest is −2.11 for Haiti.

The expected effect of government effectiveness on mask-wearing behavior is not straightforward to define. Intuitively, people in a country with high government effectiveness might be more likely to trust public policies and, therefore, follow encouraging mask-wearing announcements from their government. However, the opposite hypothesis is also possible. For example, people might not feel the need to take personal measures against the pandemic if they believe the government can contain it.

COVID-19 Case Trend (*trend*) The timing of policy implementation significantly influences its effectiveness. Since mask-wearing is a preventive measure against

COVID-19, infection trends are likely to impact how people respond to related government communications. To evaluate infection trends, this study uses the number of infections per 100,000 people, sourced from Our World in Data (Mathieu et al., 2020). The trend indicator is calculated as the ratio of the seven-day moving average of new infections at two time points: the day of SP and 7 days earlier. A value below 1 indicates a decreasing trend, while a value above 1 signifies an increasing trend.

Similar to the *ge* factor, the potential relationship between infection trends and public reactions is open to interpretation. For instance, if COVID-19 cases are already declining, citizens might feel less urgency to follow mask-wearing announcements. Conversely, they may interpret these announcements as warnings of a potential future increase in cases and adjust their behavior accordingly.

Mask-Wearing Ratio (*mask*) The impact of mask-wearing announcements could be limited if a majority of citizens are already wearing masks. The mask-wearing ratio is calculated from respondents in each dataset of Step One before the SP. It would represent the extent of this "ceiling effect."

Government Approval Rate (*approv*) Mask-wearing announcements from a popular government would be more likely to be followed. Directorio Legislativo, a private research institution based in Argentina and the United States, publishes monthly approval rates of governments in Latin America, estimated from multiple surveys (Directorio Legislativo, 2023), although there are some data gaps. This paper uses the institution's data for the month of SP. If data for that month is not available, the approval rate would be calculated as the average of the previous month's rate and the next month's rate. To ensure this estimate aligns with the general trend in approval rates, it is cross-checked with the Executive Approval Database (Carlin et al., 2023), which covers approval rates for the world's principal governments, though it has less data on Latin American countries than Directorio Legislativo. The nine cases where the approval rate could not be calculated due to missing data from the previous or next year were excluded from the fsQCA. All these cases had LATEs of zero.

Relative Acuteness of Announcement (*cos*) The potential impact of a mask-wearing announcement can be influenced by the context established by prior communications. For instance, if a government were to mandate mask-wearing without any preceding announcements on the subject, such a policy might be perceived as abrupt or unexpected. In contrast, if the government had gradually introduced mask-wearing recommendations beforehand, the mandate would likely be seen as a natural extension of existing practices. To represent the relative acuteness of announcement, as illustrated in Fig. 4.3a, an index called "cosine (*cos*)" was established. It takes into account not only the target announcement (C) but also the levels of the preceding announcements (B and A).

Cosine values of θ were computed to plot the angles within a square frame. According to the OxCGRT classification, mask-wearing announcements fall into

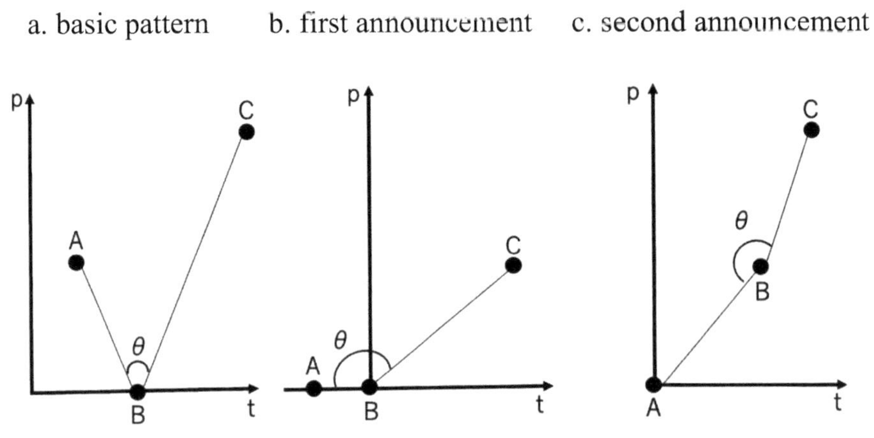

Fig. 4.3 *cos* condition (t: time, p: mask-wearing announcement level)

five levels: (0) absence of a policy, (1) recommendation to wear masks, (2) requirement to wear masks in specific shared spaces outside the home or where social distancing is impractical, (3) mandate to wear masks in all shared spaces outside the home or where social distancing is not feasible, and (4) continuous mask usage outside the home. Since the announcement changes span five stages and the study covers 838 days (between the first day of identification of the COVID-19 infection, February 20, 2020, in Mexico, and the day of the last announcement, June 7, 2022, in Mexico), the policy values were scaled by a factor of 209.5 to enable angle plotting within the square frame.

The cosine of θ approaches 1 when the duration of policy maintenance is short and the level of change is significant, while it approaches -1 when the duration of policy maintenance is long and the level of change is minimal. Using the dot product formula, the cosine of θ is calculated as:

$$\cos\theta = \frac{\overrightarrow{BA} \cdot \overrightarrow{BC}}{|BA||BC|} \tag{4.1}$$

In the case of the first announcement of a country, A is located on $(-1, 0)$ and B on the origin (Fig. 4.3b). In the case of the second announcement, A is on the origin, while B and C are located according to their values on passed days and implemented announcement level (Fig. 4.3c).

4.3.2 *Calibration*

In fsQCA, it is necessary to calibrate each condition into a continuous range from 0 to 1. The calibrated values are referred to as membership values. Except for the outcome and the trend condition with the reasons explained later, the calibration

Table 4.3 Calibration

	Description	Min	Max	Cut-off
<Outcome>				
LATE	Significant LATEs for Step One, otherwise 0	−0.020	0.114	[a]
<Conditions>				
ge	Government efficiency index of World Government Index at the year of SP	−1.889	0.850	−0.5
trend	Ratio of 7-day average of COVID-19 cases per 1,000,000 between the day of SP and that 7 days before SP	0.663	3.422	[a]
mask	Ratio of mask-wearing of the respondents before SP	0.452	0.851	0.7 0.666
approv	*Directorio Legislativo* approval rate at the month of SP	14	83	47
cos	Relative extent of announcement acuteness	−0.968	0.996	0

[a] Manual assignment

was performed using the R's QCA package, employing the direct method.[1] An overview of the calibration process is provided in Table 4.3.

For the outcome, since a LATE of 0 indicates no change in mask-wearing behavior, intuitively the cut-off threshold should be set just above 0, such as at 0.001. However, this setting results in a nuanced case distinction, assigning a membership value of 0.466, very close to 0.5, to 21 out of 29 cases with a LATE value of 0 (Fig. 4.4a). To create a clearer distinction between cases with positive LATEs and those with null or negative LATEs, the membership values are manually adjusted: cases with a positive LATE are assigned a value of 1, those with null LATE are penalized and assigned a value of 0.25, and cases with a negative LATE are assigned a value of 0.

For the conditions, the cut-off thresholds are determined to divide cases into two groups with distinct characteristics, based on the distribution of values. For *ge*, the threshold was set at −0.5 (Fig. 4.4b) for two reasons. First, when the values are arranged in descending order, this threshold corresponds to the largest difference between two adjacent values. Second, given that state capacity tends to remain stable over short periods, the groups formed by the threshold should not overlap in terms of included countries. The cut-off value of −0.5 satisfies this criterion by creating mutually exclusive groups: the positive group includes Uruguay, Chile, Costa Rica, Panama, Colombia, the Dominican Republic, Mexico, and Peru, while the negative group comprises El Salvador, Paraguay, Honduras, Bolivia, Guatemala, Nicaragua, and Venezuela.

For *trend*, the cut-off threshold of 1—representing no change in the 7-day moving average of COVID-19 cases—resulted in many cases clustering around 0.5 (Fig. 4.4c). To address this nuanced distinction, membership values were manually assigned: cases with a value above 1 were allocated a membership value of 1, while those with a value of 0 or lower were assigned 0.

---

[1] I am deeply grateful to Sho Niikawa for their valuable suggestions.

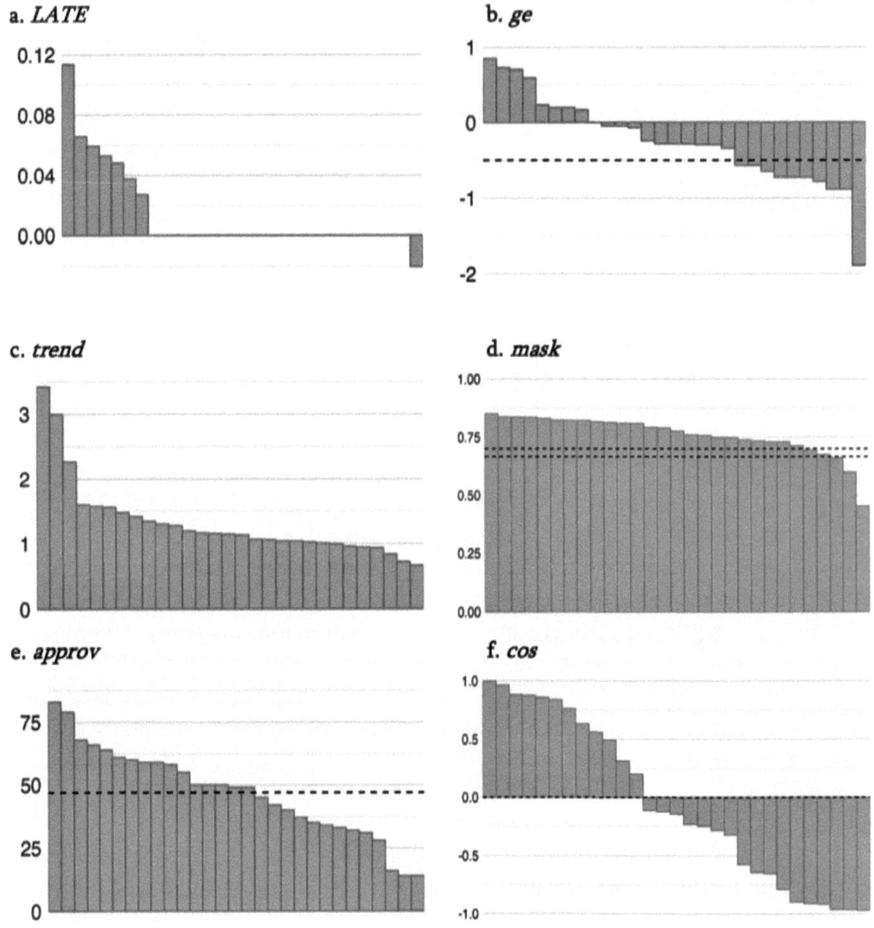

Fig. 4.4 Distribution of values across cases (dashed line: cut-off threshold)

For *mask*, identifying a threshold that signifies a saturation point in mask-wearing proved challenging. The distribution of values indicates two potential cut-off points: 0.7, which groups the five lowest cases, and 0.666 (two-thirds), which includes the three lowest cases (Fig. 4.4d). For *approv*, the threshold was set at 47, dividing cases into those with an approval rate of 50% or higher and those with a lower rate (Fig. 4.4e). Finally, the threshold for *cos* was set at 0, categorizing 12 cases as positive (Fig. 4.4f). The negative cases are referred to as additional announcements, where governments issued one or two incremental levels of mask-wearing mandates following a previous announcement that had already increased the level of compliance.

Table 4.4 Necessary conditions for positive LATEs

mask cut-off	Combination	Cons.	RoN	Cov
0.7	*~ge + ~trend + ~mask + ~approv*	0.922	0.506	0.564
0.666	*~trend + ~mask + cos*	0.901	0.528	0.517

Cons: consistency, Cov: coverage

Table 4.5 Sufficient conditions for positive LATEs

mask cut-off	Combination	inclS	PRI	covS	Case
0.7	*ge * ~ mask*	0.864	0.727	0.490	Cos200615_200705; Dom220228_220320
	*~mask * ~ approv*	0.861	0.705	0.407	Nic210209_210301
	*~ge * cos * approv*	0.829	0.608	0.418	Gua210709_210726
	*~trend * cos * ~ approv*	0.895	0.862	0.131	Chi210419_210509
0.666	*~mask*	0.914	0.830	0.485	Cos200615_200705; Nic210209_210301; Dom220228_220320
	*~ge * cos * approv*	0.829	0.608	0.418	Gua210709_210726
	*~trend * cos * ~ approv*	0.895	0.862	0.131	Chi210419_210509

4.3.3 Necessary and Sufficient Conditions

Starting with positive LATEs, the necessary conditions with a consistency above 0.9, as well as the highest relevance of necessity (RoN) and coverage, are as follows (Table 4.4):

Common combinations identified across the two sets of results obtained with different *mask* cut-offs demonstrate robustness in explaining the relationship between the outcome and the conditions. Specifically, the absence of COVID-19 case expansion (~*trend*) and a low mask-wearing ratio (~*mask*) are essential conditions for mask-wearing announcements to be effective. This suggests that people are more likely to perceive government encouragement as an alert in scenarios where there is no worsening of COVID-19 cases and where there is still room for improvement in mask-wearing rates.

The parsimonious solutions of sufficient conditions with a consistency higher than 0.75 and a proportional reduction in inconsistency (PRI) over 0.5, following the recommendation of Greckhamer et al. (2018), are as follows (Table 4.5):

These results provide three key findings. First, the absence of a high mask-wearing ratio (~*mask*) emerges as the simplest and most influential factor for effective announcements. Among the seven cases with positive LATEs, three fall into this category: Costa Rica in June–July 2020, Nicaragua in February–March 2021, and the Dominican Republic in February–March 2022. Considering the necessary condition discussed above, this finding supports the presence of a "ceiling effect" in mask-wearing announcements, wherein their effectiveness diminishes as mask-wearing rates approach saturation.

Second, the case of Guatemala in July 2021 represents a distinct path, characterized by a low level of government efficiency, an acute announcement, and a high popularity of the government. During this period, Alejandro Giammattei served as the president of Guatemala, a country historically considered as one of the least developed in Latin America (Mahoney, 2012, pp. 5–6). Despite facing a political crisis in late 2020 sparked by protests against budget cuts for vulnerable groups, including COVID-19 patients, Giammattei managed to recover politically and maintained a 59% approval rate (Directorio Legislativo, 2023). The movement of announcements issued in July 2021 recorded the highest *cos* score (0.996) among all cases analyzed in this study. On July 5, the government lifted the mask-wearing mandate, which had been in place for more than 14 months and was classified as the highest level of announcement by OxCGRT. However, the mandate was reinstated just 8 days later. This abrupt policy reversal, resembling a form of shock therapy, had a significant impact, resulting in a positive LATE.

Finally, Chile in April–May 2021 represents an additional path, characterized by the absence of COVID-19 expansion, an acute announcement, and a low approval rate. Sebastián Piñera, the country's right-wing president during this period, had experienced historically low popularity starting in November 2019, when mass protests erupted due to widespread dissatisfaction with the government's inaction on social issues. While COVID-19 case trends remained stable and public attention was largely focused on the upcoming general elections in November 2021, the government, with an approval rate below 20%, adjusted its mask-wearing mandate twice within a few months. On December 15, 2020, the mandate was relaxed from "always wear outside home" (level 4) to "wear when social distancing is impracticable" (level 2). Four months later, on April 26, 2021, the mandate was reinstated at a stricter level, requiring masks in all shared spaces (level 3). However, it should be noted that this path remains exceptional due to its lower level of coverage compared to the other conditions discussed above.

For conditions leading to negative LATEs, the analyses produced a consistent result: a high mask-wearing ratio (*mask*) emerged as the necessary condition. The following results, which meet the same criteria as those for positive LATEs, illustrate this (Table 4.6):

The sufficient conditions, also meeting the same criteria of those of positive LATEs, are the following (Table 4.7):

Two common combinations emerged across the results from different mask cutoffs: *ge* * *trend* * *mask* and *trend* * *mask* * ~ *approv*. These results suggest that two factors—an increase in COVID-19 cases (*trend*) and a high mask-wearing ratio (*mask*)—are likely to reduce the effectiveness of government encouragement for mask-wearing. This finding aligns with the results discussed earlier: mask-wearing announcements are effective as alerts only in the absence of a worsening pandemic

Table 4.6 Necessary conditions for negative LATEs

mask cut-off	Combination	Cons	RoN	Cov
0.7	*mask*	0.926	0.575	0.730
0.666	*mask*	0.967	0.507	0.720

Cons: consistency, Cov: coverage

Table 4.7 Sufficient conditions for negative LATEs

mask cut-off	Combination	inclS	PRI	covS	case
0.7	*~ge * ~ cos * approv*	0.850	0.634	0.301	3 cases
	*ge * trend * mask*	0.873	0.800	0.580	11 cases
	*trend * mask * ~ approv*	0.824	0.702	0.469	7 cases
0.666	*ge * trend * mask*	0.871	0.798	0.588	11 cases
	*trend * mask * ~ cos*	0.872	0.802	0.494	11 cases
	*trend * mask * ~ approv*	0.812	0.688	0.475	7 cases

threat, and the ceiling effect of mask-wearing limits their impact. When these factors occurred alongside either an effective government (*ge*) or a lack of government popularity (*~approv*), the combination rendered the announcement ineffective. It is worth noting that these two combinations represent different pathways toward negative LATEs: the former suggests that people governed by effective governments did not take mask-wearing promotions seriously, while the latter indicates that people under unpopular governments were less likely to follow such announcements.

4.4 Conclusion with a Special Attention to State Capacity

Government announcements related to mask-wearing can be effective, but only under very specific conditions. First, encouraging mask-wearing has the potential to be effective, whereas discouraging it does not. Second, the most critical factor influencing the success or failure of mask-wearing announcements is the mask-wearing ratio at the time the announcement is made (*mask*). The presence or absence of the ceiling effect strongly determines the effectiveness of these announcements. Third, the trend of COVID-19 cases interacts with other factors to influence the outcomes of mask-wearing announcements. Contrary to the intuitive assumption that an announcement issued during an aggravating pandemic would motivate people to wear masks, this study demonstrates that the absence of an increasing trend (*~trend*) enhances the effectiveness of announcements, while its presence (*trend*) leads to their ineffectiveness. This suggests that the message of mask-wearing announcements resonates under stable COVID-19 case trends, where people are less likely to perceive a strong threat. Finally, mask-wearing announcements can be effective when they disrupt the trend of prior announcements (*cos*), although this forms part of exceptional pathways toward positive effectiveness that include additional factors, such as government effectiveness (*ge*) and government approval rate (*approv*).

What does this conclusion contribute to the understanding of the connections among public policy, state capacity, and the COVID-19 pandemic? The disaggregation of state capacity (Okada, Chap. 1) and the mapping of various public policies (Akiyoshi et al., 2017; Hughs, 2018) provide a foundation for exploring the characteristics of mask-wearing announcements. This volume stipulates that state capacity can be divided into two aspects: coercive and coordinative. The coercive aspects involve the government's ability to impose policies through bureaucratic resources. These include the direct provision of goods and services, such as primary healthcare (Masukata, Chap. 5), vaccine rollouts (Okada, Chap. 3; Sanmartín & Bortz, Chap. 8), and pandemic relief payments (Bizberg, Chap. 2), as well as the enforcement of behavioral restrictions, such as travel bans, stay-at-home orders, and prohibitions on large gatherings. On the other hand, the coordinative aspects highlight communication between governmental and non-governmental actors in the policy-making process, such as in collaborative governance (Bianchi et al., Chap. 7).

Mask-wearing announcements occupy a unique position within this framework. First, these announcements are generally informational measures intended to guide public behavior in ways deemed desirable by the government. While certain mandates may include penalties for non-compliance, most announcements lack coercive elements and do not require the mobilization of extensive public resources. Second, these announcements did not result from intensive communication between the government and civil society. Instead, decisions on announcements were often made by a small policy circle comprising bureaucrats from ministries responsible for health issues and external experts, relying on knowledge from international organizations such as the Pan American Health Organization/World Health Organization[2] (Vargas, 2020; Portal, 2022).

This low presence of both coercive and coordinative aspects means that announcements regarding mask-wearing have very weak leverage to change public behavior. Their success, therefore, depends on public voluntaristic decision to follow them. This character aligns well with the results of this chapter's analysis, in which government effectiveness (*ge*), the proxy of state capacity, did not appear frequently as a condition both for effective and ineffective announcements.

However, the results also provide two intriguing insights regarding state capacity. First, the observed causal direction of *ge* on effectiveness is negative: its absence (~*ge*) formed part of a sufficient condition for effective announcements, while its

[2] The decision-making process for public alerts has not been thoroughly examined (Sadiq et al., 2023: 1732–1733), including mask-wearing policies in Latin America. This chapter speculates that the exclusivity of these decisions arises from the broad scope of their target audience and the urgency of the situation. Unlike policies directed at specific groups, mask-wearing announcements target the general public. Governments also needed to address the uncertainties surrounding COVID-19 while avoiding prolonged deliberations. Given the difficulty of defining a unified public will and managing unexpected situations, issuing such announcements from a limited decision-making circle may have been deemed the most practical approach.

presence (*ge*) contributed to ineffective ones. This finding suggests that high state capacity does not necessarily guarantee voluntary behavioral change among the public. On the contrary, high state capacity could undermine the effectiveness of mask-wearing announcements. This implies that encouraging or mandating mask-wearing functions less as a reflection of public trust or obedience toward well-established governments and more as an alert that prompts individuals in contexts of precarious public services to adopt self-protective measures. Second, the limited role of *ge* in significant conditions indicates that any government, regardless of its level of state capacity, has the potential to issue effective announcements. Recognizing the ceiling effect and understanding public perception of announcements as preemptive alerts are crucial for issuing announcements at an appropriate time.

This chapter examined mask-wearing announcements in Latin America as a policy case that challenges the intuitive connection between high state capacity and strong performance in addressing COVID-19-related issues. The relationship between the two is not straightforward. Those engaged in public administration for pandemics should consider the specific characteristics of a policy and its interaction with state capacity to achieve the desired outcomes when planning and implementing interventions.

Acknowledgments This research is based on results from the University of Maryland Social Data Science Center Global COVID-19 Trends and Impact Survey, in partnership with Facebook, and was supported by JSPS KAKENHI Grant No. 20KK0024. I am grateful to Isamu Okada, Hirokazu Kikuchi, and Shuichiro Masukata for their valuable comments during meetings related to this study. I also appreciate the participants of the panel "State Capacity and COVID-19 in Latin America" of the International Political Science Association, held on July 19, 2023, at Universidad Católica Argentina, and the International Workshop "Comparative Perspectives on State Capacity and the COVID-19 Pandemic in Latin America," held on March 22, 2024, at El Colegio de México, for their fruitful comments and insightful discussions, which helped me map perspectives for analyzing public policies related to COVID-19 in the context of Latin America. Finally, I would like to express my special gratitude to Sho Niikawa and Andreas Corcaci for their suggestions, which enhanced my analysis presented at the 4th Japan Workshop on Qualitative Comparative Analysis, held on September 3, 2024, at Waseda University.

References

Akiyoshi, T., Ito, S., & Kitayama, T. (2017). Kokyo Seisaku Gaku no Kiso (Foundations of policy studies (revised edition.). Yuhikaku.

Boulos, L., Curran, J. A., Gallant, A., Wong, H., Johnson, C., Delahunty-Pike, A., Saxinger, L., Chu, D., Comeau, J., Flynn, T., Clegg, J., & Dye, C. (2023). Effectiveness of face masks for reducing transmission of SARS-CoV-2: a rapid systematic review. *Philosophical Transactions of the Royal Society A, 381*(2257). https://doi.org/10.1098/rsta.2023.0133

Brüssow, H., & Zuber, S. (2022). Can a combination of vaccination and face mask wearing contain the COVID-19 pandemic? *Microbial Biotechnology, 15*(3), 721–737.

Callaghan, T., Lueck, J. A., Trujillo, K. L., & Ferdinand, A. O. (2021). Rural and urban differences in COVID-19 prevention behaviors. *The Journal of Rural Health, 37*(2), 287–295.

Capraro, V., & Barcelo, H. (2020). The effect of messaging and gender on intentions to wear a face covering to slow down COVID-19 transmission. arXiv preprint arXiv:2005.05467.

Carlin, R. E., Hartlyn, J., Hellwig, T., Love, G. J., Martinez-Gallardo, C., & Singer, M. M. (2023). Executive Approval Database 3.0. Retrieved December 15, 2024, from https://executiveapproval.org/download/.

Cohen, J. (1989). *Statistical power analysis for the behavioral sciences* (2nd ed.). Lawrence Erlbaum Associates.

Directorio Legislativo. (2023). Presidential approval data in Latin America, according to a new edition of the "Image of Power" report. Retrieved August 20, 2024 from https://directoriolegislativo.org/en/presidential-approval-data-in-latin-america-according-to-a-new-edition-of-the-image-of-power-report/.

Greckhamer, T., Furnari, S., Fiss, P. C., & Aguilera, R. V. (2018). Studying configurations with qualitative comparative analysis: Best practices in strategy and organization research. *Strategic Organization, 16*(4), 482–495.

Haischer, M. H., Beilfuss, R., Hart, M. R., Opielinski, L., Wrucke, D., Zirgaitis, G., Uhrich, T., & D., & Hunter, S. K. (2020). Who is wearing a mask? Gender-, age-, and location-related differences during the COVID-19 pandemic. *PLoS One, 15*(10), e0240785.

Hale, T., Angrist, N., Goldszmidt, R., Kira, B., Petherick, A., Phillips, T., Webster, S., Cameron-Blake, E., Hallas, L., Majumdar, S., & Tatlow, H. (2021). Oxford COVID-19 government response tracker (OxCGRT). *Nature Human Behaviour.* https://doi.org/10.1038/s41562-021-01079-8

He, L., He, C., Reynolds, T. L., Bai, Q., Huang, Y., Li, C., et al. (2021). Why do people oppose mask wearing? A comprehensive analysis of US tweets during the COVID-19 pandemic. *Journal of the American Medical Informatics Association, 28*(7), 1564–1573.

Hearne, B. N., & Niño, M. D. (2021). Understanding how race, ethnicity, and gender shape mask-wearing adherence during the COVID-19 pandemic: evidence from the COVID impact survey. *Journal of Racial and Ethnic Health Disparities*, 1–8.

Hughs, O. (2018). *Public management and administration: An introduction* (5th ed.). Red Globe Press.

Imbens, G. W., & Lemieux, T. (2008). Regression discontinuity designs: A guide to practice. *Journal of Econometrics, 142*(2), 615–635.

Mahoney, J. (2012). *Colonialism and postcolonial development: Spanish America in comparative perspective.* Cambridge University Press.

Mathieu, E., Ritchie, H., Rodés-Guirao, L., Appel, C., Gavrilov, D., Giattino, C., Hasell, J., Macdonald, B., Dattani, S., Beltekian, D., Ortiz-Ospina, E., & Roser, M. (2020). COVID-19 pandemic. Retrieved June 29, 2023, from: https://ourworldindata.org/coronavirus.

Miyachi, T. (2023). The short-term impact of central government announcements on mask-wearing behavior in Latin America: An analysis of Meta COVID-19 Survey Data. Paper presented at 27th World Congress of Political Science, Universidad Católica Argentina, July 19.

Palmer, C. L., & Peterson, R. D. (2020). Toxic Mask-ulinity: The link between masculine toughness and affective reactions to mask wearing in the COVID-19 era. *Politics & Gender, 16*(4), 1044–1051.

Papageorge, N. W., Zahn, M. V., Belot, M., Van den Broek-Altenburg, E., Choi, S., Jamison, J. C., & Tripodi, E. (2021). Socio-demographic factors associated with self-protecting behavior during the Covid-19 pandemic. *Journal of Population Economics, 34*, 691–738.

Pew Research Center. (2020). Republicans, democrats move even further apart in coronavirus concerns. Retrieved December 31, 2024, from https://www.pewresearch.org/politics/2020/06/25/republicans-democrats-move-even-further-apart-in-coronavirus-concerns/.

Portal, J. Á. (2022). Respuesta de Cuba para enfrentar la COVID-19 y sus retos. *Revista Cubana de Medicina Tropical, 74*(3) Retrieved December 31, 2024, from https://revmedtropical.sld.cu/index.php/medtropical/article/download/973/641

Rieger, M. O. (2020). To wear or not to wear? Factors influencing wearing face masks in Germany during the COVID-19 pandemic. *Asian Journal of Social Health and Behavior, 3*(2), 50–54.

Rihoux, B., & Ragin, C. (2008). *Configurational comparative methods: Qualitative comparative analysis (QCA) and related techniques.* Sage Publications.

Sadiq, A. A., Okhai, R., Tyler, J., & Entress, R. (2023). Public alert and warning system literature review in the USA: Identifying research gaps and lessons for practice. *Natural Hazards, 117*(2), 1711–1744.

Sakakibara, R., & Ozono, H. (2021). Hitobito ga Masuku wo Chakuyo Suru Riyu Towa: Kokunai Kenkyu no Tsuishi to Risachi Kuesuchon no Kensho (Why do people wear a mask? A replication of previous studies and examination of two research questions in a Japanese sample). *The Japanese Journal of Psychology, 92*(5), 332–338. in Japanese.

Vargas, M. (2020). Diplomacia científica: El rol del científico en el manejo de pandemias. *Revista de Bioética y Derecho, 50*, 255–270.

World Bank. (2023). Worldwide governance indicators. Retrieved June 29, 2023, from https://info.worldbank.org/governance/wgi/.

Xu, K. L. (2017). Regression discontinuity with categorical outcomes. *Journal of Econometrics, 201*(1), 1–18.

Yang, L., Constantino, S. M., Grenfell, B. T., Weber, E. U., Levin, S. A., & Vasconcelos, V. V. (2022). Sociocultural determinants of global mask-wearing behavior. *Proceedings of the National Academy of Sciences, 119*(41), e2213525119.

Chapter 5
Path-Dependent Disparities of Brazil's Healthcare System and State Response in Coping with COVID-19

Shuichiro Masukata

5.1 Introduction

This chapter argues that the long-term structural inequalities embedded in Brazil's healthcare system—rooted in colonial legacies and reinforced by neoliberal reforms—have shaped the path-dependent disparities in the state's capacity to implement primary healthcare policies. These disparities, in turn, conditioned the country's uneven and inadequate response to the COVID-19 pandemic. By tracing the institutional evolution of the Unified Health System (Sistema Único de Saúde, SUS) and examining its response to the pandemic, this chapter highlights how historical legacies continue to influence the efficacy and equity of healthcare delivery in times of crises.

The COVID-19 pandemic in 2020 caused severe damage worldwide, and Latin America was among the regions with the highest number of COVID-19 infections and deaths. People within and outside Latin America criticized the World Health Organization (WHO) for its inability to lead global infectious disease control and universal health coverage (UHC) efforts. However, the WHO's International Health Regulations only require scrutinizing countries' quarantine standards and healthcare services. Therefore, the response to past global infectious disease pandemics, such as severe acute respiratory syndrome (SARS) and novel influenza (H1N1 2009), was ultimately left to the judgment of individual countries (Clinton & Devi, 2017).

In short, the weaknesses of global health governance have created a situation in which the ability to respond adequately to the spread of infectious diseases depends on state capacity and public policies. For this book, state capacity is defined as "the capacity to implement its decisions over society effectively" (Okada, Chap. 1). Following this definition, the adequate functioning of primary healthcare

S. Masukata (✉)
Keio University, Tokyo, Japan
e-mail: s-masukata@keio.jp

I. Okada (ed.), *COVID-19 and State Capacity in Latin America*, Latin American Societies, https://doi.org/10.1007/978-3-032-15572-6_5

(PHC) systems during emergencies also depends on the degree of professional organization and the country's capacity to provide administrative services, which is defined as state capacity. In general, PHC is widely recognized as the most appropriate way to provide access to the health system and is directly associated with a more equitable distribution of health among populations (Fernandez et al., 2024a, 2024b).

While the global COVID-19 pandemic has been addressed through proactive national frameworks, this study aims to identify how Brazil's healthcare system responded to the COVID-19 pandemic. The healthcare system in Latin American countries has mainly pursued the political aims that dominate their relations with government and civil societies (Dalton and Weatherford, eds., 2022). Brazil, however, is the only country in Latin America to have introduced UHC in the 1980s and has a highly regarded SUS that aims to achieve UHC. The adoption of SUS has been explained in the past as increased state accountability for the demands of the popular health movement during democratization (Gibson, 2019). Notably, the PHC policy was regulated by the National Primary Care Policy (Política Nacional de Atenção Básica, PNAB), first introduced in 2006 and revised in 2012 and 2017 under the SUS. The PNAB governs the scope of actions to be provided by PHC, the types of services subsidized by the federal government, and the responsibilities of the federated entities regarding the care level (Ministério da Saúde, 2023). Hence, PHC policy in Brazil is responsible for PHC for the Brazilian population through health promotion, palliative care, and health surveillance within the SUS.

For better or worse, Brazil has received the most attention for its response to COVID-19 through its primary health system. The existing literature is filled with criticisms of the state's diminishing role due to neoliberal reforms since the 1990s (Duarte, 2023; Machado & Lima, 2024). Neoliberalism has powerfully impacted at least five dominant factors in the healthcare sector: politics, finance, professional activity, institutional governance mechanisms, and citizens' entitlements and choices. These have become major drivers of rising healthcare costs (Benatar et al., 2020, p. 446). Hence, previous studies have criticized the state's diminishing role due to neoliberal reforms since the 1990s, which weakened PHC and exacerbated the damage caused by COVID-19 (Farias et al., 2022; Duarte, 2023; Machado & Lima, 2024). In contrast, positive arguments also exist that the health sector's institutional resilience was maintained despite the neoliberal reforms. Resilience in healthcare is defined as the diverse capacities of a healthcare system that allow it to support the delivery of high-quality care after events that challenge, disrupt, enhance, or reorganize system functioning in response to those events (Wiig et al., 2020).

However, these arguments have not yet adequately answered the three questions of this book. This study analyzes the innovation of healthcare policy and assesses the implementation and outcomes of SUS in coping with the COVID-19 pandemic. To foreshadow the conclusions of this chapter, PHC's institutional outcomes in SUS while dealing with the COVID-19 pandemic, which is one of the indicators of Brazil's state capacity, can be significantly attributed to historically sedimented institutional and fiscal inequalities. Historical inequalities in Brazil's health system have led to many limitations regarding regional and social inequalities, creating disparities in national capacity and, consequently, health outcomes such as mortality during the COVID-19 pandemic.

This study makes two significant contributions to the literature. First, the form of government and the implementation of the state's response to problems such as infectious diseases are constrained by the enduring mechanisms of disparities. Thus, the PHC was forced into a limited reaction to the COVID-19 pandemic crisis. Second, the remaining challenges in responding to COVID-19 highlight the need for a more effective institutional framework for implementing healthcare policies. The progress and obstacles in building universal health institutions in Brazil—one of the world's largest economies but with stark regional and social inequalities—are shaped by social, economic, and regional disparities, which also negatively affect the performance of the primary healthcare system.

The remainder of this chapter is organized as follows. Section 5.2 shows how the existing literature failed to examine path dependency regarding primary healthcare systems. Section 5.3 proposes a research design for examining path-dependent disparities in primary healthcare. Section 5.4 applies this perspective to analyze the path dependency of historical inequality in the healthcare system in Brazil. Section 5.5 discusses the effectiveness of the healthcare system in implementing COVID-19 countermeasures and highlights gaps in responding to the pandemic. Section 5.7 concludes with policy and theoretical implications.

5.2 Historical Path Dependency and Primary Healthcare Systems

Previous research on implementing state public policies has produced significant literature on path dependence (Pierson, 2000, 2004). The concept of path dependence, initially developed in economics, has recently gained traction in comparative politics and sociology as a valuable analytical tool for understanding political and social phenomena. Researchers increasingly employ this framework to dissect how past events and decisions shape present-day realities, moving beyond static analyses to incorporate a dynamic understanding of social processes. Paul Pierson, a prominent scholar in this area, emphasizes the importance of temporality in social inquiry. He aims to "explicate different ways in which things happen over time in social life, drawing attention to processes that are unlikely to be visible without specifically addressing questions of temporality" (Pierson, 2004, p. 10). In essence, Pierson argues that many crucial social dynamics are missed when time and historical sequence are not explicitly considered.

Pierson posits that the political sphere is particularly susceptible to self-reinforcing behavior, a concept synonymous with positive feedback, path dependence, and increasing returns (Pierson, 2000). He suggests that once a particular course of action is adopted in politics, it becomes increasingly challenging to deviate from it, even if more efficient or desirable alternatives emerge later. This tendency is not random; rather, it stems from inherent characteristics of the political realm that amplify the influence of initial choices. In the healthcare context, despite UHC expansion, the SUS faces organizational and governance challenges, inadequate funding, and poor resource allocation. These structural problems will likely worsen and risk reversing the institution's achievements in improving outcomes. Although path dependency focuses primarily on formal political institutions, this approach does not exclude the analysis of other factors that explain collective or individual behavior. From this concept, path dependency is used to analyze public policy. While many studies conceptualize path dependency as driven by increasing returns or self-reinforcing sequences (Pierson, 2000), this chapter also draws attention to reactive sequences in which institutional legacies constrain new policy choices without necessarily producing functional efficiency (Mahoney, 2010). This view allows us to analyze how historically unequal institutional arrangements in Brazil's health system have imposed limits on recent policy innovations and pandemic response.

In contrast, the broad literature on state responses to COVID-19 sheds light on health policies in the context of national systems, such as the SUS, and how countries take different paths at critical junctures (Twigg, 2020; Hajnal et al., 2021). In the Brazilian health system, Massuda et al. (2024) address investment policies for PHC in SUS through a historical lens. Investment policies are vital for how a health system is set up, especially in the Brazilian SUS, where PHC plays a key role. They emphasize why funding PHC is essential and how that funding affects the results. Ultimately, this helps us understand PHC, considering the historical context and the factors that have influenced it (Castro et al., 2019; Dimas, 2022; Navai, 2022).

Additionally, the key components of healthcare system resilience include governance and leadership, financing, resources (workforce, infrastructure, medicines, and technology), and service delivery (Wharton & MacGuire, 2024). Fernandez et al. (2024a, 2024b) found that poor leadership and governance hindered the system's performance. Yet, despite the challenges, the system was able to offer care and carry out a successful vaccination initiative. Their study also highlighted how factors like governance, federal arrangements, and social participation help maintain and adapt the system. Simultaneously, they identified weaknesses such as funding, decentralization, and inadequate human resources, which limited the system's ability to adapt to the crisis (Fernandez et al., 2024a, 2024b).

While existing studies may explain SUS's contributions and limitations, the literature has yet to adequately explain how the measures against COVID-19 are connected to the historical restrictions that have persisted in the SUS. Therefore, path dependence is the most appropriate theoretical foundation for analyzing state capacity and the outcomes of PHC implementation, which is this study's objective. This chapter describes how historical inequality has led to disparities in coping with COVID-19 (disparities in state capacity and resulting health outcomes). Assessing the consequences of SUS healthcare policy is directly linked to Brazil's state capacity to respond to COVID-19.

5.3 Research Design: Path-Dependent Disparities in Primary Healthcare

To understand how the COVID-19 pandemic updates the meaning of state capacity, I must closely examine the historical long-term factors that have enabled or constrained it. This study argues that path-dependent disparities shaped how a state leveraged professional organizations to enhance its state capacities and implementation outcomes in response to COVID-19.

This chapter explains the path dependence of disparity using four facets. The first is the disparity in antecedent conditions. These disparities precede and shape a diverse set of features in the economy, society, and politics that establish the parameters for subsequent changes. The origins of political, economic, and social disparities in Latin America trace back to the colonial period (Mahoney, 2010; Sanchéz-Ancochea, 2021). The political systems of the colonies were deeply intertwined with class systems. Large landowners were able to exercise substantial influence and power, shaping political systems and policies that served their own interests while suppressing the influence and rights of Indigenous groups and enslaved people. Latin American countries experienced transformations even before gaining independence in the nineteenth century. By the late nineteenth century, a series of technological innovations made international trade easier and cheaper, rapidly expanding the export of primary products. Inequality was exacerbated by traditional systems and strong economic elites established during the colonial period (Sanchéz-Ancochea, 2021, p. 24).

The second is the disparity in implementation regarding the SUS prior to the COVID-19 pandemic. Brazil's SUS is based on the principle that all Brazilian citizens and foreigners living in Brazil have universal access to healthcare services, regardless of economic class or gender. The SUS was established on the principle defined in the 1988 federal constitution: health is a universal right and a responsibility of the state. It is regulated by federal law and implemented at the federal, state, and municipal levels, which enjoy political, financial, and administrative autonomy. The SUS is a decentralized public health system that coexists with a private health insurance sector that supplements public services. Government responsibility is shared between three levels—federal, state, and municipal—with political, financial, and administrative autonomy.[1]

Moreover, the SUS includes mechanisms for social participation at all levels of government and is open to private sector involvement. Despite chronic underfunding for over 30 years, the SUS has successfully expanded access to healthcare services, mainly through the Family Health Strategy and PHC policy (Castro et al., 2019). Recognized internationally, SUS serves as a model for universal health care initiative worldwide (Lindelow, 2013).

[1] Brasil (1990) Law No. 8080 regulates conditions for the promotion, protection and recovery of health, the organization and operation of corresponding services and other measures. Presidency of the Republic, Brasflia. http://www.planalto.gov.br/ccivil_03/Leis/L8080.htm.

With the SUS's introduction, over 150 million people—approximately 75% of the Brazilian population—became procedurally eligible for the primary care program. However, even before the outbreak of the COVID-19 pandemic, implementation disparities caused by regional and socioeconomic inequalities persisted (Massuda et al., 2018).

The third is the disparity caused by neoliberal reforms since the SUS was introduced. Latin American countries implemented neoliberal reforms in the 1990s in response to the debt crisis. Many governments in the region embarked on neoliberal market reforms, with state-controlled entities, such as public health systems, being sold to private companies. Proponents of neoliberalism argued that privately managed, market-driven systems would expand coverage, reduce costs for patients, and better adapt to local needs through competition (Dimas, 2022, p. 288). Neoliberal reforms have allowed Latin American countries to reform their states to become more efficient. However, these initiatives conflicted with universal health principles and exacerbated regional and socioeconomic inequalities, which in turn contributed to health disparities.

In sum, the historical gap exacerbated disparities in coping with COVID-19. From 2020 to the present, the COVID-19 pandemic forced Latin American countries—already shaped by neoliberal reforms since the 1990s—to respond using their existing healthcare systems. Institutional responses and their effectiveness varied across countries due to path dependencies within these systems.

To identify how the above three factors combined to exacerbate disparities in responses to COVID-19, I surveyed news articles, statistics, and other data published by international and governmental sources, along with primary and secondary scholarly materials. In recent decades, seven countries in Latin America and the Caribbean (LAC-7: Argentina, Chile, Colombia, Costa Rica, Peru, Mexico, and Brazil) have made significant efforts to strengthen their primary healthcare systems. On multiple occasions, other Latin American countries also pursued proactive primary healthcare policies. The effective functioning of health systems has contributed substantial economic and social benefits to these nations (OECD, 2022, p. 3). While this chapter focuses on Brazil as a single case study, the analytical approach can be applied to other Latin American contexts.

5.4 Historical Disparities in the Healthcare System in Brazil

This case study illustrates how path-dependent disparities in Brazil's healthcare system influenced its response to the COVID-19 pandemic. Generally, path dependence is a long-term factor that remains resilient over time. Capacity is built path-dependently in the sense that a political choice at one-point extracts resources and uses them for institution-building in a specific sphere, creating an underlying baseline for future policy implementation. The characteristics of Brazil's healthcare system in its 2020 pandemic response provide valuable insights into measuring path-dependent disparities over a sufficient temporal distance. This subsection disaggregates the disparities in Brazil's pandemic response into three categories—healthcare infrastructure, fiscal investment, and health outcomes—each reflecting distinct forms of path-dependent inequality embedded in the country's institutional trajectory.

5.4.1 Disparities in Antecedent Conditions: State Capacity

In 1937, the Brazilian Ministry of Education and Public Health was renamed. That same year, the government launched the National Yellow Fever Control Program, the first public health program at the national level. From the 1930s to the 1980s, Brazil experienced state-led industrialization—mainly through import substitution industrialization and rapid urbanization. Urbanization led to significant demographic changes. While Brazil's national mortality and fertility rates declined and life expectancy increased, state formation exacerbated the disparity between urban and rural areas.

The state formation period can be divided into two phases. The first was the period of Getúlio Vargas' dictatorship (*Estado Novo*) and the subsequent populist administrations from the 1930s to the 1960s. One notable example is the first Vargas administration, during which conservative, liberal, and military governments vied for leadership and initiated programs to transform the country or preserve the status quo.

Under the Vargas administration, public health developed as a centralized government program. The federal government initiated annual national medical conferences to showcase these reforms. A key step in restructuring the public health system was the creation of a program called the Federal Health Delegation. The Brazilian health system was characterized by a public health program based on a social insurance model, emphasizing infectious disease control and medical support services for urban workers in the formal sector (Dimas, 2022).

5.4.2 Disparities in Antecedent Conditions: Beyond State Capacity

Multiple antecedent conditions shaped disparities in Brazil's healthcare system. The first is social conditions. Most of the country lies in the tropics, making it highly vulnerable to infectious diseases. Therefore, analyzing the formation of Brazil's healthcare system is tantamount to exploring the development of a centralized government structure. The Brazilian government could not afford to underestimate the importance of infectious diseases in citizens' lives. From the period of modern nation-building around 1930 to the present, the country has faced several endemic diseases, including yellow fever, leprosy, malaria, and Chagas disease.

The second is political authority. Starting in the 1930s, health policy was shaped by two primary factors: government efforts to combat easily transmitted diseases, and health services for formal workers under a social insurance model (Fonseca, 2007). In the early years of the military regime (1965–1969), the government systematized Brazil's healthcare under the National Health Policy (Paim et al., 2011). During this period, approximately 95% of children received vaccination coverage, and vaccines were relatively inexpensive due to domestic production. The military regime defined Brazil's national health system, centralized financial control under social security institutions, and empowered technical bureaucracies to manage the growing commercialization of health services (Lima, 2005; Falleti, 2010). The link between health and democracy later emerged through the strengthening of the democratic movement, including the health reform movement (Movimento da Reforma Sanitária), which opposed the military regime in the mid-1970s social and political context.

5.4.3 SUS and Implementation: Institutional Design Configuration

The SUS emerged from the 1988 Constitution in the name of universality and equity (Barbara, 2018). The system is inclusive, accessible, and universally available to all Brazilian citizens, regardless of economic or social status (Machado & Silva, 2019, p. 15). The Constitution also established the broader concept of social security encompassing healthcare, pensions, social assistance, and UHC, which guarantee comprehensive care for the population.[2]

The SUS operates under a complex governance structure that necessitates collaborative management across federal, state, and municipal levels. This multi-tiered approach is crucial for ensuring equitable access across Brazil's vast and diverse regions. At the federal level, the Ministry of Health plays a central role, exerting significant influence through its seven executive secretariats. These secretariats are responsible for formulating national health policy and program guidelines, impacting everything from disease prevention to hospital infrastructure.[3]

Beyond the internal structure of the Ministry, the National Health Council (Conselho Nacional de Saúde, CNS), a vital advisory body, provides external guidance. The CNS plays a key role in advising the Ministry of Health on the definition and prioritization of health initiatives, ensuring that policy decisions are informed by a broad range of perspectives and address the most pressing needs of the population. Complementing the Ministry and the CNS are several other significant entities linked to the Ministry, each with specialized functions. The National Health Agency (Agência Nacional de Saúde, ANS) is responsible for regulating private health

[2] Brasil. Ibid.

[3] Brasil. Ibid.

insurance plans, while the National Health Surveillance Agency (Agência Nacional de Vigilância Sanitária, ANVISA) is tasked with ensuring the safety and efficacy of pharmaceuticals, medical devices, and food products. The Oswaldo Cruz Foundation (Fundação Oswaldo Cruz, Fiocruz) serves as a renowned research institution dedicated to advancing public health through scientific innovation and technological development. Additionally, the National Committee for Technology Incorporation (Commissão Nacional de Incorporação de Tecnologias, Conitec) is responsible for evaluating and incorporating health technologies into the SUS.[4]

The Ministry of Health spearheaded the initial implementation of SUS, carefully defining municipal responsibilities and establishing the financial mechanisms needed to sustain the system. This framework laid the foundation for the decentralized structure that still characterizes SUS today (Machado & Lima, 2024, pp. 729–730).

Since the 1990s, strong federal leadership has been instrumental in ensuring coordination across the SUS. It has helped consolidate relatively uniform health policies across the country despite enduring regional disparities rooted in socioeconomic and geographic inequalities (Massuda et al., 2018; Machado & Lima, 2024).

The following sections explore the institutional arrangements that support Brazil's national health system, highlighting the collaborative governance between government entities and providers from both public and private sectors. Understanding this interplay is crucial to appreciating the challenges and possibilities of delivering universal healthcare in Brazil.

5.4.4 SUS and Implementation: Implementation Disparities

Despite its achievements, SUS implementation has always been marked by disparities. The massive expansion of Brazil's healthcare system includes both public and private facilities. The most significant growth occurred in primary care services—health centers and family health units—more than 99% of which are public. This suggests improved access to publicly provided primary healthcare. Private clinics and polyclinics have also grown, most either contracted under private health insurance or operating independently. In terms of hospitals, some new municipal facilities have opened, but private hospitals continue to dominate—many serving both SUS and private clients. Diagnostic and therapeutic support services are primarily private and serve both sectors. This illustrates how public and private healthcare systems in Brazil are deeply interconnected (Machado & Silva, 2019, p. 15).[5]

[4] Brasil. Ibid.

[5] Private healthcare sector has expanded and diversified with the SUS relying on private providers. High private spending, exceeding 50% of total healthcare spending, contradicts the universal public system. This spending is primarily on health plans and out-of-pocket expenses, especially for low-income families buying medicines. The dynamism of private markets, fueled by subsidies,

5.4.5 Fragmented Responses During the Pandemic

Governments continued these policies, but from 2003 to 2016, the Workers' Party (Partido dos Trabalhadores, PT) administration counteracted some negative effects of earlier reforms. Redistributive welfare programs during this period were associated with higher incomes, lower unemployment, and reduced inequality.

This favorable political and economic environment enabled increased public funding for the SUS, improving access to essential services for nearly all Brazilians and reducing regional health disparities. Nevertheless, health inequities persisted (Massuda et al., 2018).

Massuda et al. (2018) examined SUS's post-2000 growth and the economic and political crises that began in 2014, along with subsequent austerity measures and their impact on SUS. External and internal shocks such as economic and political crises result in job losses, poverty, and cuts in healthcare spending, forcing people to seek help from social support programs. This cascade of events affects people's healthcare behavior and outcomes, leading to unfair differences in health. Political and economic crises undermine social programs and UHC policies. The Michel Temer administration, which succeeded the PT government, implemented a neoliberal economic agenda that included the privatization of major state-owned assets. In 2016, Congress passed Constitutional Amendment 95 (EC95/PEC55/PEC241), capping federal primary expenditures on health for 20 years. Financing reforms targeted specific PHC components, while national health policies were revised to promote private insurance options, reduce public sector demand, and introduce low-cost plans with limited benefits (Doniec et al., 2016). SUS had to respond to the Zika virus and other emerging diseases under these increasingly restrictive conditions.

Proponents of neoliberalism argue that privately managed, market-driven systems improve coverage while reducing and tailoring costs. However, citizens still rely heavily on state-run systems, and many professionals and experts warn that privatization may worsen an already precarious situation (Dimas, 2022). Indeed, disparities in access, inadequate public funding, and worsening health outcomes persisted and deepened during Brazil's democratic recession.

5.5 The Disparity in Managing the COVID-19 Pandemic

The COVID-19 pandemic has become a benchmark for assessing the health outcomes of Brazil's healthcare system. Primary healthcare (PHC) in SUS is the country's longest-running healthcare system. In February 2020, the COVID-19 epidemic broke out in Brazil, causing enormous damage to an economy that was showing

---

creates competition for resources, hindering the consolidation of the SUS and reducing health inequalities (Machado & Lima, 2024, p. 730).

signs of recovery. This included corporate bankruptcies, loss of jobs and income, and a worsening fiscal balance. As political and social divisions surfaced, the Bolsonaro administration, which had come to power the previous year, embraced neoliberal reforms, including privatization, tariff cuts, and social security and tax reforms. This administration reflected the enduring legacy of the neoliberal critical juncture in SUS's response to COVID-19. PHC played a crucial role in reducing the pandemic's impact, preserving and expanding characteristics of SUS such as accessibility to initial contact, long-term individual care, comprehensive care, care coordination, cultural competence, and a focus on families and communities (Daumas et al., 2020, p. 2).

5.5.1 Political Institutions, State Capacity, and Crisis Management

The COVID-19 crisis exposed deep-rooted disparities in PHC that pose a serious threat to public health. Neoliberal policies created a divided and fragmented healthcare system in which wealthy minorities can access advanced private healthcare, while most of the population depends on a severely underfunded public system. This makes the public health system a less desirable option for low-income individuals.

Decision-making and implementation based on intergovernmental coordination are factors that measure state capacity. In contrast, the decentralization promoted by SUS in the face of COVID-19 also revealed widening regional and economic disparities that have long challenged Brazil. The Brazilian government failed to consider that socioeconomically vulnerable states were at high risk of being overburdened by COVID-19, and the functionality of health systems in these states declined. Especially in the nation's northeastern and northern regions, where the socioeconomic situation was already fragile, health system budgets and implementation were inadequate, and the damage caused by COVID-19 was generally more severe. In addition, the lack of adequate federal planning to improve the health system's resilience increased existing health disparities in the country.

Brazil's government underestimated COVID-19's impact on socioeconomically vulnerable states, leading to poorer health system performance in those regions. This lack of planning to improve resilience resulted in a significant decrease in healthcare procedures and exacerbated the country's existing health disparities (Bigoni et al., 2022).

5.5.2 Disparities in Health Outcomes

As mentioned above, Brazil has established health and social systems. Despite this, COVID-19 spread rapidly in Brazil and led to clear disparities in health outcomes.

Infrastructure Disparities: Uneven Health System Capacity

Table 5.1 reveals stark regional inequalities in healthcare infrastructure, such as ICU beds and medical personnel. For example, the North and Northeast regions had only 4.3 and 5.7 SUS ICU beds per 100,000 people, respectively, compared to 8.9 in the South. These disparities reflect historical underinvestment in peripheral regions, rooted in the legacies of centralized development and urban-centric health policies initiated during Brazil's industrialization and military regimes (cf. Sects. 5.4.1 and 5.4.2). Such path-dependent inequalities in infrastructure limited the responsiveness of health systems in poorer states, making these areas more vulnerable during the pandemic.

Fiscal Disparities: Budget Allocation and Capacity to Respond

Beyond infrastructure, fiscal disparities also shaped Brazil's uneven response to COVID-19. Table 5.1 shows that regions with higher vulnerability indexes—especially the North and Northeast—had lower per capita investments in new ICU beds during the early phases of the pandemic.

These discrepancies can be traced to Brazil's federal fiscal architecture, which decentralizes health responsibilities to states and municipalities without ensuring equitable transfers. Despite SUS's universalist aspirations, fiscal autonomy—exacerbated by Constitutional Amendment 95 (EC95)—has allowed disparities to persist or deepen (cf. Sect. 5.4.5). The results suggest that state capacity is path-dependently unequal, shaped by a mismatch between decentralization and redistributive mechanisms.

Outcome Disparities: Mortality and Exposure to COVID-19

Outcome indicators, such as age-adjusted COVID-19 deaths per 100,000 people, reveal the compounded effects of infrastructure and fiscal inequalities. As of October 2020, death rates were highest in the North (99.9) and Northeast (79.4), and lowest in the South (45.4).

The mortality rates from COVID-19 reflect these compounded effects. According to Rocha et al. (2021), the North had the highest mortality rates despite attempts at stricter measures. These path-dependent outcome disparities emerge from overlapping vulnerabilities—underfunded healthcare, weak municipal capacity, and historical exclusion from welfare expansion. Outcome indicators—such as age-adjusted COVID-19 deaths per 100,000 people—reveal the compounded effect of infrastructure and fiscal inequalities. As of October 2020, death rates were highest in the North (99.9) and Northeast (79.4), and lowest in the South (45.4). Rocha et al. (2021) highlight that municipalities with high socioeconomic vulnerability initially enacted stricter policy responses but still experienced worse outcomes due to entrenched inequalities. This reinforces the view that historical structural disparities

Table 5.1 Inequalities in socioeconomic characteristics, health system resourses, and governmental response in Brazil and its regions (authors' adaptation)

		Average by region				
	Brazil	North	Northeast	Center-west	Southeast	South
COVID-19 deaths per 100,000 people, age-adjusted (as of Oct 31, 2020)	76.2	99.9	79.4	90.2	85.9	45.4
Socioeconomic vulnerability						
Socioeconomic vulnerability index	0.62	0.79	0.8	0.44	0.33	0.31
Housing vulnerability (%)	44.5	56.8	50.1	44.6	19.8	32
Informal workers (%)	25.7	29.8	26.9	24.4	22.4	19
Health vulnerability						
Population with health risk factors (%)	47	43.2	45.7	49	50.3	52.9
Population aged >60 years (%)	16.1	12.7	17.2	15.4	19.2	18
Pre-existing hospital services						
SUS ICU beds per 100,000 people	6.1	4.3	5.7	6.5	8	8.9
Private ICU beds per 100,000 people	9	2.8	4.4	31.6	10.1	5.5
ICU physicians per 100,000 people	15.2	7.2	11.4	22.9	24	23.1
Pre-existing primary healthcare and social assistance						
Community health agents' coverage (%)	72.4	78.1	86	59.7	56	56.7
Family health strategy coverage (%)	72.1	69.9	84.7	63	59.3	68.7
Bolsa família coverage (%)	8	8.7	12.6	4.1	4.5	2.8
Response and outcomes as of June, 2020						
New ICU beds (per 100,000 people)	4.4	3.6	4.7	4.8	3.7	5.2
New ICU beds (% of pre-existing)	82.9	108.2	88.5	77.3	48.7	60.2
Policy stringency index	53.4	54	57.5	40.6	57.8	50.9
Change in physical distancing adherence since February, 2020 (percentage points)	10.8	11	12	9.4	10.2	9.8
COVID-19 deaths per 100,000 people, age-adjusted	31.8	50.2	34.2	11.3	34.5	5.1
Response and outcomes as of October, 2020						
New ICU beds (per 100,000 people)	7.3	5.3	7.1	9.3	8.3	9.2
New ICU beds (% of pre-existing)	130.2	142.2	131.3	147.6	105.1	108.9
Policy stringency index	37	40	33.6	43.8	27.7	43.2
Change in physical distancing adherence since February, 2020 (percentage points)	6.5	5.8	8.2	5.5	5.9	4.9

Credit: Adapted from *The Lancet Global Health*, 9(6), Rocha R, Atun R, Massuda A, **et al.** (2021), "Effect of socioeconomic inequalities and vulnerabilities on health-system preparedness and response to COVID-19 in Brazil: a comprehensive analysis," e782–e792, **Table, with permission from Elsevier.** © 2021 The Author(s). Published by Elsevier Ltd. doi: 10.1016/S2214-109X(21)00081-4

in public service provision, healthcare access, and informal labor markets played a decisive role in worsening the pandemic's impact.

Thus, Brazil's pandemic mortality map reflects a path-dependent geography of vulnerability, shaped by colonial land inequality, incomplete welfare expansion, and uneven institutional development.

5.6 Discussion: Path-Dependent Disparities to Primary Healthcare in Times of Crisis

This chapter's analysis of Brazil's case shows that historical disparities led to disparities in coping with COVID-19. The implementation disparities demonstrated that gaps in national capacity in responding to the COVID-19 pandemic and the worsening consequences of responses were accelerated. These disparities were not incidental but reflected deeply rooted institutional patterns shaped by colonial legacies and reinforced by neoliberal reforms. This chapter demonstrated that such path-dependent disparities constrained the state's ability to deliver an equitable and effective pandemic response.

It highlights the increase in the healthcare budget since the reforms and the worsening of existing challenges. Over the past years, the SUS has been impacted by neoliberal reforms advocated by the World Bank, which criticized the constitutional guarantee of universal healthcare and promoted private sector involvement in service delivery (Massuda et al., 2018). Comprehending the organization and movement of healthcare spending is crucial for evaluating the components of financial resilience. Since the establishment of the SUS, its funding has been inadequate.

This budget increase occurred during the Rousseff administration from 2011 to 2016. President Rousseff, who succeeded in implementing the Lula administration's policies, aimed to expand social security for low-income groups. However, she cut the healthcare budget at the beginning of her administration. The budget increased following massive demonstrations in Brazil in 2013, and this trend intensified after the Temer administration took office in September 2016, in what was described as a shift toward neoliberal reforms.

A further increase was observed in the 2019–2020 health budget of the Bolsonaro administration (Fig. 5.1). The increase, even before the outbreak of the COVID-19 pandemic, might be evidence of the system's durability. However, under Temer (2016–2018), and especially Bolsonaro (2019–2022), public health governance was based on political clientelism and market-privatizing interests, with the adoption of long-term fiscal austerity policies, deepening privatization, and SUS defunding (Chioro et al., 2023). Furthermore, a survey conducted in 2019 indicated that more than 70% of the population had no access to healthcare services.

This study also shows that the response to the COVID-19 pandemic did not correct the severe regional and health disparities in the Brazilian population (Bigoni et al., 2022).

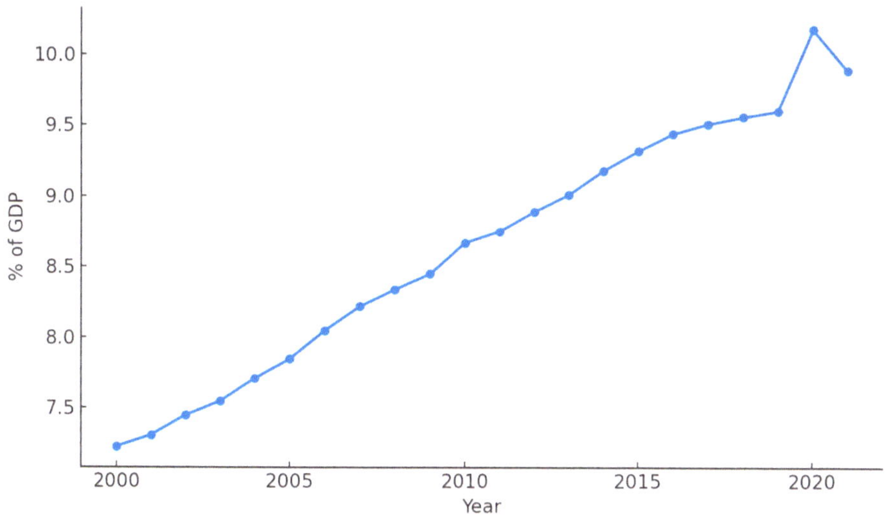

Fig. 5.1 Brazil-current health expenditure (% of GDP), 2000–2021. Source: Authors' visualization based on *World Bank, World Development Indicators* (indicator **SH.XPD.CHEX.GD.ZS**), Brazil, 2000–2021, accessed [28 Oct 2025]. **License:** CC BY 4.0

5.7 Conclusion

Importantly, this chapter illustrates that path dependency is not only a constraint on reform but also a structuring force for institutional resilience. In Brazil, the SUS has shown signs of adaptability through community-level responses and professional commitment despite structural inequalities. However, resilience remains uneven and incomplete where historical disparities in capacity have gone unaddressed. Thus, path-dependent trajectories can shape both the vulnerabilities and the adaptive strengths of state institutions.

The COVID-19 pandemic amplified and brought to light a problem that had not been previously visualized. This study analyzed historically dependent disparities in the implementation and outcomes of the SUS. The progress in building universal institutions in Brazil that has continued thus far has been essential in increasing state capacity. Still, the inadequate outcomes in implementing these institutions and measures are defined by the structural problems that have persisted over the long term.

This consideration stems from states' responses to the COVID-19 pandemic. In addition to exposing inequalities and devastating public health, the government's reaction to the pandemic has had dangerous repercussions in Brazil, exacerbating socioeconomic inequality and democratic recession. While decentralization can widen regional disparities, it can also enable grassroots solutions to national-level shortcomings. Additionally, it highlights the value of healthcare professionals who are invested in the system and policies, as they can use their expertise to challenge political decisions.

This chapter's findings have crucial implications when combined with historical and institutional factors. First, path dependency provides a valuable way to explain the extent of state institutions' professional organization and broad changes in administrative services without being able to fully resolve social disparities. The path-dependent inequalities of the primary healthcare system became evident during the COVID-19 pandemic. Many governments have made efforts to correct the systemic disparities inherent in the SUS. Although some corrections were made in the 2000s, they did not go far enough to solve the fundamental problem, and the systems that promote socioeconomic disparities continue to reinforce themselves. Additionally, the SUS presents a fundamental challenge that must be acknowledged. The Brazilian government must address and correct socioeconomic disparities, such as regional and class disparities, and ensure equitable budget allocation for healthcare regardless of pandemic emergencies. In Brazil, municipalities are unequal in degrees of capacity. These high inequalities among municipalities in terms of state capacities jeopardize resilience in the face of crisis.

Comparative experiences from Mexico and Argentina during the COVID-19 pandemic further underscore how institutional legacies shaped state responses. In Mexico, centralized federal control and limited vertical coordination weakened local adaptability despite strong scientific leadership. Conversely, Argentina leveraged a more cooperative model of intergovernmental governance, with active social participation, enabling a relatively more unified national response. While all three countries faced constraints, Brazil's path-dependent decentralization without equitable fiscal equalization mechanisms made regional disparities more entrenched. These cases collectively highlight that not only institutional design but also the historical pathways through which such designs evolve affect pandemic resilience.

Second, this study provides the possibilities of structural explanations for the distinct evolution of Latin American healthcare systems. While it traced the historical institutional change and the healthcare system in Brazil, the case can provide various lessons in Latin America as a whole. Specifically, comparative historical analyses of health systems in Brazil and other Latin American countries, such as Mexico, will likely prove applicable to other Latin American contexts (Bizberg, Chap. 2). Attention to antecedent conditions helps clarify how institutional settings shape both change and continuity, as well as how turning points influence how different types of institutions develop. The pandemic responses in Mexico and Argentina were supported by factors such as governance, federalism, and social participation, which demonstrate the state's capacity to maintain and adapt the health system. However, as in Brazil, vulnerabilities such as unequal funding distribution, decentralization, and lack of human resources limited the ability to adapt to the crisis. The findings from Brazil suggest that path-dependent disparities are not merely legacies of the past but active structures that shape institutional resilience and state capacity in present-day crises. Comparative studies across Latin America may benefit from examining how different historical legacies and reform trajectories have conditioned pandemic responses.

Acknowledgments This work was supported by JSPS KAKENHI Grant Numbers 20KK0024, 21H04392, and 23H00041. The author would like to express his gratitude to the Oswaldo Cruz Foundation and Butantan Institute in Brazil. However, the author is responsible for the wording of the article.

References

Barbara, V. (2018, December 11). Brazil's new president isn't even in office yet, and he's already damaged health care. *The* New York Times. https://www.nytimes.com/2018/12/11/opinion/brazil-health-care-bolsonaro.html.

Benatar, S., David, S., & Gill, S. (2020). The global politics of health care reform. In C. McInnes, K. Lee, & J. Youde (Eds.), The Oxford handbook of global health politics (pp. 445–468). Oxford University Press.

Bigoni, A., Malik, A. M., Tasca, R., Carrera, M. M., Schiesari, L. C., Gambardella, D. D., & Massuda, A. (2022). Brazil's health system functionality amidst the COVID-19 pandemic analysis of resilience. *The Lancet Regional Health-Americas, 10*, 100222.

Castro, M. C., Massuda, A., Almeda, G., et al. (2019). Brazil's unified health system: The first 30 years and prospects for the future. *The Lancet, 394*(10195), 345–356.

Chioro, A., Temporão, J. G., Massuda, A., et al. (2023). From Bolsonaro to Lula: The opportunity to rebuild universal healthcare in Brazil in the government transition. *The International Journal of Health Planning and Management, 38*(3), 569–578. https://doi.org/10.1002/hpm.3627

Clinton, C., & Devi, L. S. (2017). *Governing global health: Who runs the world and why?* Oxford University Press.

Daumas, R. P., Azevedo e Silva, G., Tasca, E., et al. (2020). The role of primary Care in the Brazilian healthcare system: Limits and possibilities for fighting COVID-19. *Cadernos de Saúde Pública, 36*(6). https://doi.org/10.1590/0102-311X00104120

Dimas, C. S. (2022). Health as a right in Brazil and Argentina. In D. S. Dalton & D. J. Weatherford (Eds.), *Healthcare in Latin America: History, society, culture* (pp. 278–295). University of Florida Press.

Doniec, K., Dall'Alba, R., & King, L. (2016). Austerity threatens universal health coverage in Brazil. *The Lancet, 388*(10047), 867–868.

Duarte, A. (2023). *Pandemic and crisis of democracy: Biopolitics, neoliberalism, and Necropolitics in Bolsonaro's Brazil.* Routledge.

Farias, D. B. L., Casarões, G., & Magalhães, D. (2022). Radical right populism and the politics of cruelty: The case of COVID-19 in Brazil under president Bolsonaro. *Global Studies Quarterly*. https://doi.org/10.1093/isagsq/ksab048

Falleti, T. (2010). Infiltrating the state: The evolution of health care reforms in Brazil; 1964-1988. In J. Mahoney & K. Thelen (Eds.), *Explaining institutional change: Ambiguity, agency, and power* (pp. 38–62). Cambridge University Press.

Fernandez, M., Massuda, A., & Tasca, R. (2024a). Reaffirming primary health care's vital role. *The Lancet, 403*(10435), 1448–1449.

Fernandez, M., Paschoalotto, M. C., Lotta, G., et al. (2024b). Resilience in the Brazilian health system: Impacts of the COVID-19 pandemic. In S. Thomas & P. Freming (Eds.), *Handbook of health system resilience*. Elgar Publishing.

Fonseca, C. M. O. (2007). *Saúde no Governo Vargas (1930–1945): Dualidade institucional de um bem público*. Editora Fiocruz.

Gibson, C. L. (2019). *Movement-driven development: The politics of health and democracy in Brazil.* Stanford University Press.

Hajnal, G., Jeziorska, I., & Kovács, E. M. (2021). Understanding drivers of illiberal entrenchment at critical junctures: Institutional response to COVID-19 in Hungary and Poland. *International Review of Administrative Sciences, 87*(3), 612–630.

Lima, N. T. (org.) (2005). Saúde e Democracia: história e perspectivas do SUS. Editora Fiocruz.
Lindelow, M. (2013). The hallmark of the Brazilian National Health System. *World Bank Group* (https://www.worldbank.org/en/news/opinion/2013/12/20/brazil-sus-unified-public-healthcare-system-new-study) Assessed to 20 July, 2025.
Machado, C. V., & Silva, G. A. E. (2019). Political struggles for a universal health system in Brazil: Successes and limits in the reduction of inequalities. *Globalization and Health, 15*(Suppl. 1), 77.
Machado, C. V., & Lima, L. D. (2024). Brazil's unified health system: The fight for a universal right in an unequal country. *Salud Publica Mexicana, 66*, 726–731.
Mahoney, J. (2010). *Colonialism and development: Spanish America in comparative perspective*. Cambridge University Press.
Massuda, A., Hone, T., Leles, F. G., de Castro, M. C., & Rifat, A. (2018). The Brazilian health system at crossroads: Progress, crisis, and resilience. *BMJ Globalization and Health, 3*(e000829). https://doi.org/10.1136/bmjgh-2018-000829
Massuda, A., Fernanda, M., & Paschalotto, M. A. (2024). Analysis of investment policies in primary health care: Historical neo institutionalism applied to the Brazilian health system. *Brazilian Journal of Public Administration, 58*(2), e2023–e0391. https://doi.org/10.1590/0034-761220230391x
Ministério da Saúde (2023). Portal da Secretária da Atenção Primaria a Saúde (Saps). https://aps.saude.gov.br/smp/smpoquee.
Navai, P. C. (2022). SUS: uma reforma revolucionária: para defender a vida. Autêntica.
OECD. (2022). *Primary health care for resilient health systems in Latin America. OECD health policy studies*. OECD Publishing. https://doi.org/10.1787/743e6228-en
Paim, J., Travassos, C., Almeida, C., Bahia, L., & Macinko, J. (2011). The Brazilian health system: History, advances, and challenges. *Lancet, 377*(9779), 1778–1797.
Pierson, P. (2000). Increasing returns, path dependence, and the study of politics. *The American Political Science Review, 94*(2), 251–267.
Pierson, P. (2004). *Politics in time: History, institutions, and social analysis*. Princeton University Press.
Rocha, R., Atun, R., Massuda, A., et al. (2021). Effect of socioeconomic inequalities and vulnerabilities on health-system preparedness response to COVID-19 in Brazil: A comprehensive analysis. *Lacet Global Health, 9*(6), e782–e792. https://doi.org/10.1016/S2214-109X(21)00081-4
Sanchéz-Ancochea, D. (2021). *The costs of inequality: Lessons and warnings for the rest of the world*. Bloomsbury.
Twigg, J. (2020). COVID-19 as a 'Critical Juncture': A scoping review. *Global Policy, 2020*, 1–20.
Wharton, G., & MacGuire, A. (2024). Assessing health system sustainability and resilience: Reporting on the partnership for health system sustainability and resilience (PHSSR). In S. Thomas & P. Freming (Eds.), *Handbook of health system resilience* (pp. 73–88). Elgar Publishing.
Wiig, S., Aase, K., Billett, S., et al. (2020). Defining the boundaries and operational concepts of resilience in the resilience in healthcare research program. *BMC Health Service Research, 20*(330). https://doi.org/10.1186/s12913-020-05224-3

Chapter 6
State Capacity and Policy Diffusion in Latin America: The Case of COVID-19

Hirokazu Kikuchi

6.1 Introduction

Latin America became one of the epicenters and experienced a sharp increase in the number of cases and deaths from COVID-19. Facing this situation, governments in the region took a variety of non-pharmaceutical measures. A trend in COVID-19 policy-making in Latin America was the heavy use of presidential decrees based on the declaration of a state of emergency. Legislatures met only a few times during the initial period of the pandemic, as holding such meetings was a potential risk factor for generating infection clusters. As a result, the legislative branches in Latin American countries approved few measures for the economy, public health, and travel restrictions, most of which were implemented via presidential decrees.

Holding the implementation channel as a constant, the fact that we observed a variety of measures taken by countries in Latin America is puzzling. González-Bustamante (2021) showed that fiscal expenditure on health, decentralization, and pressure on the health system led to stringent interventions in the early stage of the pandemic in South America. Based on the case studies on Brazil and Peru, Cameron et al. (2023) argued that the preparedness of the health system influenced perceived political risks, which led Vizcarra and Bolsonaro to take different measures.

A solution to understand this puzzle is to analyze the relationship between state capacity and diffusion. On the one hand, some studies attributed the high death toll to the weak state capacity of countries in the region such as Peru (Knutsen & Kolvani, 2024). On the other hand, some studies found homogeneity in the declaration of a state of emergency in Latin America, suggesting regional policy diffusion among policymakers in non-pharmaceutical interventions (Lundgren et al., 2020). Therefore, this chapter asks the following questions: Did state capacity play a crucial role in the diffusion of non-pharmaceutical interventions in Latin America? If

H. Kikuchi (✉)
Institute of Developing Economies, Japan External Trade Organization, Chiba, Japan
e-mail: hirokazu_kikuchi@ide.go.jp

I. Okada (ed.), *COVID-19 and State Capacity in Latin America*, Latin American Societies, https://doi.org/10.1007/978-3-032-15572-6_6

so, which dimension of state capacity did matter? The heavy use of presidential decrees in the region during the pandemic provides a unique opportunity to study the relationship between state capacity and policy diffusion. One difficulty in studying this relationship is that policies are usually implemented through various channels. However, in the case of the COVID-19 pandemic, most policies were implemented via presidential decrees, which enables us to study the impacts of state capacity on policy diffusion (especially via emulation) through their comparisons. In addition, we could isolate emulation from other mechanisms of policy diffusion because of the prompt need to take non-pharmaceutical interventions without knowing the intervention results of other countries.

In this chapter, I argue that emulation patterns in the texts of presidential decrees were related to some dimensions of state capacity. State capacity consists of extractive capacity, administrative capacity, and coercive capacity (Hanson & Sigman, 2021). It is expected that a similar level of administrative and coercive capacities led a pair of two countries to issue similar decrees, because structural equivalence in a social network, which can be interpreted as socioeconomic similarity, facilitates emulation (Maggetti & Gilardi, 2016; Yi & Liu, 2022), and administrative capacity (Cronert, 2022; González-Bustamante, 2021) and coercive capacity (Ganga & Schenk, 2024) were the main determinants of non-pharmaceutical interventions in the literature. It is also expected that policymakers tended to imitate the texts of decrees issued by a country with a high administrative capacity, and that a country with a lower administrative capacity tended to imitate the texts of decrees issued by other countries. I test the validity of these arguments by combining a dyadic approach in the study of policy diffusion (e.g., Hinkle, 2015; Düpont & Rachuj, 2022) with a text analysis of presidential decrees issued in 12 countries between February and March in 2020. This chapter directly addresses one of the questions of this book ("What do state strengths and weaknesses explain about the responses and outcomes to the COVID-19 pandemic?"), while the findings of the chapter have implications for the other two questions.

The argument of this chapter is developed as follows. I review the literature of social science studies on the role of state capacity in the case of COVID-19, paying attention to multi-dimensions of state capacity. I then develop hypotheses that connect such multi-dimensions of state capacity with policy diffusion of measures against COVID-19. To test my hypotheses, I conduct a text analysis to generate the dependent variable. Finally, I conduct statistical tests for the two types of hypotheses and discuss each result.

6.2 Multi-Dimensions of State Capacity

State capacity is a concept with multiple dimensions as argued in the introduction to this book, and most studies on state capacity have only focused on some of the dimensions according to their research questions. To study the success of elite taxes for public safety in Latin America, Flores-Macías (2022) focused on public safety and fiscal extraction following Weber's (1978) argument that the state holds a monopolistic power over legitimate violence in a territory. In analyzing state building in Latin America, Kurtz (2013) did not highlight such Weberian logic. He instead paid attention to the strength of the institutions of public administration based on Mann's (1993) idea of infrastructural power. In an introductory chapter of the book on states in developing countries, Centeno et al. (2017) also claimed that organizational capacity is the only dimension that influences a state's performance. According to them, resources, the presence of the state in its societies, the professionalization of the civil service, and inter- and intra-institutional communication and oversight represent the organizational capacity of the state.

Although the literature on state capacity considers seven different dimensions as a whole (Cingolani, 2013),[1] Hanson and Sigman (2021) considered extractive capacity, coercive capacity, and administrative capacity as the principal dimensions indispensable to the functioning of modern states. Extractive capacity is related to a state's ability to collect taxes, which is critical for various types of state activities, whereas coercive capacity is associated with a state's ability to protect its borders and maintain order. Administrative capacity refers to a state's organizational ability to develop and implement public policies.

Naturally, several social science studies on COVID-19 have regarded administrative capacity as a determinant of states' responses and outcomes. For example, Serikbayeva et al. (2021) used the Government Effectiveness (GE) indicator of the Worldwide Governance Indicators as a proxy of state capacity and showed that higher GE led to lower COVID-19 deaths per confirmed cases. Cronert (2022) also operationalized administrative capacity by GE and found that higher GE was associated with more delay in implementing school closures. By contrast, Knutsen and Kolvani (2024) used V-Dem's "impartial and rule-following administration" indicator,[2] which measures the degree to which public administration is biased or arbitrary (Coppedge et al., 2024), to capture state capacity. According to them, the impartial administration indicator had a positive impact on the underreporting of COVID-19 deaths,[3] and the impacts of democracy and state capacity were complementary.

Some works have also relied on subdimensions or multiple indicators of administrative capacity. González-Bustamante (2021) studied three subdimensions of administrative capacity to study the adoption of stringent interventions in South America: delivery, coordination, and analysis. He measured delivery capacity using current health expenditure per capita and coordination capacity using V-Dem's division of power index, which captures the autonomy of local and regional

[1] These seven dimensions include coercive/military, fiscal, administrative/implementation, transformative or industrializing, relational/territorial coverage, legal, and political dimensions.

[2] It is currently named as "rigorous and impartial public administration" (v2clrspct).

[3] Knutsen and Kolvani's (2024) models actually showed that the number of government-reported deaths increased as the impartial administration indicator increased, but considered that such positive correlation was due to the fact that states with higher capacity tend to be more democratic where underreporting is less likely to occur.

governments (Coppedge et al., 2024). For the analysis capacity, he used the number of COVID-19 cases, the number of hospital beds per 1000 citizens,[4] and his original burden index.[5] He concluded that health expenditure, local and regional government capacity, and pressures on the health system led South American countries to adopt suppression strategies. To demonstrate the resilience of regional health governance in Central America and its weakness in South America during the pandemic, Agostinis and Parthenay (2021) considered the indicators of resources and presence of the state such as domestic general government health expenditure per capita, external health expenditure as a percentage of total health expenditure, the number of doctors per 10,000 people, the number of hospital beds per 10,000 people, and the antiretroviral therapy coverage among people living with HIV.

Although the interests in administrative capacity dominate studies on the role of state capacity in the case of the COVID-19 pandemic, the other dimensions are not necessarily irrelevant. Croissant and Hellmann (2023) argued that coercive capacity is also important, especially where administrative capacity and people's trust are low because the government had to rely on the military and the police to introduce social distancing and curfews. Ganga and Schenk (2024) tested the role of coercive capacity during the pandemic by combining cross-national studies with subnational analysis in the case of Russia. They used military expenditures, the number of military personnel per 1000 people, and the number of police officers per 1000 people as indicators of coercive capacity, whereas they considered the number of doctors per 1000 people, the number of hospital beds per 1000 people, and government health expenditures as a percentage of GDP, and Brambor et al.'s (2020) information capacity index indicators to capture health and information capacities, which can be regarded as subdimensions of administrative capacity. Their analysis showed that a higher coercive capacity leads to a lower likelihood of implementing mask policies and restrictions on business and a greater likelihood of implementing school restrictions.

6.3 Policy Diffusion and State Capacity

In addition to state capacity, social science studies on COVID-19 have focused on policy diffusion due to widespread non-pharmaceutical interventions. Policy diffusion is the process by which prior policy choices in one unit (e.g., countries, subnational states, and cities) influence policy choices in another unit (Maggetti & Gilardi, 2016). Hereafter, I will call the former unit as *sender* and the latter unit as *receiver*. Policy diffusion generally occurs by adopting an innovation of neighboring senders because mechanisms that promote such adoption include economic competition

[4] Some studies treated the number of COVID-19 cases and the number of hospital beds per 1000 people as control variables.

[5] It is calculated as the number of confirmed cases*0.15 divided by the number of ICU beds*0.25.

among neighbors and imitation of a sender's policy (Shipan & Volden, 2008). In the case of COVID-19 policies, Lundgren et al. (2020) found a regional concentration of countries declaring a state of emergency and argued that a country's decision is influenced by other states in the same region through emulation and learning. Sebhatu et al. (2020) also found that the prior adoption of a COVID-19 policy among proximate countries in the OECD region led to the adoption of the same policy.

Social science studies on COVID-19 have acknowledged the importance of state capacity and policy diffusion in the decision to take non-pharmaceutical action. However, the current state-of-the-art methods in these studies have two shortcomings. First, the studies on state capacity and policy diffusion have not addressed each other. Indeed, some analyses on the role of state capacity (e.g., Tosun, 2023) include regional dummies to capture some regional characteristics in non-pharmaceutical policies, while studies on policy diffusion tend to regard state capacity indicators, such as the number of hospital beds per 1000 people, as control variables (e.g., Sebhatu et al., 2020). However, little attention has been paid to the relationship between state capacity and policy diffusion, even though it is natural to assume that similarities and differences in state capacity play a crucial role in the diffusion of non-pharmaceutical actions against COVID-19 if policy diffusion does occur.

Second, the literature on policy diffusion has failed to address diffusion mechanisms in the case of the COVID-19 pandemic. Studies on policy diffusion (e.g., Shipan & Volden, 2008; Maggetti & Gilardi, 2016) have identified three mechanisms: learning, emulation (imitation), and competition.[6] Learning refers to the process by which policymakers learn from policy adoption by other governments and observe its consequences, whereas emulation is adopting a policy of other governments without considering its consequences. Competition means that policymakers decide by paying attention to the economic effects of adoption by other governments to attract external resources (Shipan & Volden, 2008). Each mechanism leads to different expectations in explaining adoption patterns of non-pharmaceutical policies, but the literature (e.g., Lundgren et al., 2020; Sebhatu et al., 2020) only focused on geographical proximity and did not distinguish between mechanisms.

Some studies on state capacity have argued that narrowing the focus at the very first stage of the pandemic allows them to isolate the influence of state capacity on responses against COVID-19 from the policy diffusion effect (e.g., Yen et al., 2022). In contrast, I argue that focusing on the very first stage of the pandemic allows us to study the impact of state capacity on policy diffusion via emulation, because governments were forced to take non-pharmaceutical actions without knowing the consequences of other governments' policies due to the emergency situation.[7]

[6] Shipan and Volden (2008) also added coercion as the fourth mechanism.

[7] Lesch and Millar (2022) also argued that high levels of urgency lead to (bounded) emulation, even though they also considered that high problem uncertainty leads to learning. If we consider the other stages of the pandemic, we should take into account learning and competition as well.

How did state capacity facilitate the diffusion of non-pharmaceutical actions against COVID-19? More specifically, how did state capacity lead two countries in Latin America to have similar presidential decrees? Maggetti and Gilardi (2016) helped identify the indicators related to emulation. According to them, students of policy diffusion have considered six indicators related to the three mechanisms: geographic proximity, joint membership in some groups, success of policy, structural equivalence in a network, number of previous adopters, and trade flows. Among these indicators, the number of previous adopters is exclusively related to emulation, whereas structural equivalence is related to emulation and competition. However, the number of previous adopters does not identify what kinds of norms or policies are more likely to be adopted, and we can omit the possibility of competition at the very first stage of the pandemic. Thus, this study focuses on structural equivalence.

Structural equivalence, a term in social network analysis, means that two nodes have ties to the same third parties. These two nodes are expected to have similar characteristics and tend to imitate each other because individuals are especially influenced by those they consider similar (Borgatti & Grosser, 2015). In this vein, Yi and Liu (2022) measured this concept by socioeconomic similarity of two units such as absolute difference in economic vitality indexes, which are based on 11 indicators for demographics, economics, human and social capital, and infrastructure in 310 U.S. cities.[8] As the discussion in the previous section shows administrative capacity (e.g., Cronert, 2022; González-Bustamante, 2021) and coercive capacity (e.g., Ganga & Schenk, 2024) play a role in the adoption of non-pharmaceutical measures, the following hypotheses should be considered:

H1a: Presidential decrees on COVID-19 policies tended to be similar if issued in countries with similar levels of administrative capacity.
H1b: Presidential decrees on COVID-19 policies tended to be similar if issued in countries with similar level of coercive capacity.

Which countries were more likely to be senders and receivers of emulations in COVID-19 policies? The key assumption here is information heuristics. Zhang and Zhu (2019) hypothesized that provinces with higher economic levels tend to be imitated by those with lower economic levels in China because economic growth is the most important indicator in the country, and policymakers simply use the indicator for heuristic inference. Studying tax policy-making in Ontario and British Columbia, Lesch and Millar (2022) argued that a meso-level indicator of bounded emulation is the receivers' limited resources. In the case of emulation of COVID-19 policies, these arguments lead to the following hypotheses:

H2a: Presidential decrees on COVID-19 policies issued by senders tended to be similar to those issued by receivers if the senders' administrative capacity was high.

[8] They regarded structural equivalence as a concept that is related to competition.

H2b: Presidential decrees on COVID-19 policies issued by senders tended to be similar to those issued by receivers if the receivers' administrative capacity was low.

6.4 A Text Analysis

To test the hypotheses introduced in the previous section, I conducted statistical analyses based on presidential decrees on COVID-19 in Latin American countries issued between February and March, 2020. Focusing on the very early stage of the pandemic is essential for isolating the emulation mechanism of policy diffusion from the other mechanisms. One challenge in conducting such an analysis is the availability of data. Due to the limited online availability of the texts of presidential decrees, this study focuses on 12 out of the 20 Latin American countries.

Although the texts of presidential decrees in Brazil are available online, this study does not consider them because of the difficulty of comparing texts across different languages. For example, Leonisio and Strijbis (2012) showed that the Spanish and Basque versions of the texts of parliamentary debates generated different statistical results.[9] Thus, the focus of this study is limited to Spanish-speaking countries.

Table 6.1 summarizes the presidential decrees used in this study. Among these decrees, Decree 4 of Chile, which declared a sanitary alert, was the only one issued in February (February 5). The number of decrees in February and March ranged from 2 (Mexico) to 44 (Colombia). However, the small number of presidential decrees does not necessarily mean that the government was not interested in taking action against COVID-19. Such governments tended to implement measures via ministerial resolutions, whereas Colombia and Argentina introduced a variety of measures via presidential decrees.

I took advantage of the websites of the official gazette, legislations and regulations, congressional libraries, or the president's office of each country to collect the text data of presidential decrees (See Table 6.4 in Appendix). Mexico, Costa Rica, Colombia, Bolivia, Chile, Argentina, and Uruguay publish the text data online, whereas Guatemala, Panama, Dominican Republic, Peru, and Paraguay upload PDF files of presidential decrees. Since the only available data are scanned images for Guatemala, Panama, and Paraguay, I also used an OCR technique to convert the images into text data.

There are several ways to measure the text similarity of a pair of documents. In this study, I relied on cosine similarity, which has been used in many studies (e.g.,

[9] Recent developments in machine translation may overcome such a problem. Using machine translation for comparing party manifestos of 16 countries, Düpont and Rachuj (2022) argued that machine translation is acceptable, because machine translation and full-text translation allowed them to detect same patterns.

Table 6.1 Presidential decrees used for the analysis of this study

Country	Number of decrees	Format
Mexico	2	Text data
Guatemala	3	PDF (OCR required)
Costa Rica	12	Text data
Panama	7	PDF (OCR required)
Dominican Republic	5	PDF
Colombia	44	Text data
Peru	19	PDF
Bolivia	11	Text data
Chile	8	Text data
Paraguay	13	PDF (OCR required)
Argentina	22	Text data
Uruguay	13	Text data

Presidential decrees on COVID-19 policies issued between February and March in 2020. Sources: See Table 6.4 in Appendix

Düpont & Rachuj, 2022). The bag-of-words approach does not consider the word order and assumes that words in a document appear independently. In this approach, each word is identical to a dimension in the data space and each document is regarded as a vector that consists of non-negative values in each dimension (Huang, 2008). Using the information on the frequency of each word, we can calculate the pairwise similarity of two documents as the cosine of the angle of two vectors (Huang, 2008; Han et al., 2012). If there is no similarity between the two documents, the two vectors are orthogonal, and the value of the cosine is 0. If two documents are completely identical, the value of the cosine is 1 because the angle of the two vectors is 0.

I conducted a text analysis to calculate the cosine similarity for each pair of presidential decrees. After collecting 159 presidential decrees of 12 countries described in Table 6.1, I preprocessed the corpus of decrees by removing punctuation, numbers, symbols, URLs, separators, and function words (stop words). I also lowercased the corpus because my analysis does not require me to distinguish "Covid" from "COVID," stemmed words in the text to count words such as "sanitario" and "sanitaria" as the same, and included 4-grams to distinguish between "medidas," "sanitarias," and "medidas sanitarias." I also excluded infrequently used terms that appeared less than 1% in the corpus (Düpont & Rachuj, 2022).

This tokenization led me to generate a document term matrix and used the quanteda package of R to calculate the cosines for each pair of presidential decrees. The cosines ranged from 0.008 (between Decree 42,332 of Costa Rica and Decree 3442 of Paraguay) to 0.876 (between Decree 317/2020 and Decree 301/2020 of Argentina).

6.5 Testing H1

To test H1a and H1b, I estimated several OLS models. The concept of policy diffusion itself assumes a dyadic relationship between two governments, and it is natural to study presidential decrees on COVID-19 using dyads as the units of analysis. Since this study is interested in policy diffusion across countries, I excluded the cases in which decrees issued by the same president constitute a dyad. The N of this analysis thus came to 10,733.

The dependent variable of this study was *cosine*, which was obtained from the text analysis in the previous section. Since I excluded the cases in which a dyad contained decrees in the same country, this variable ranged from 0.008 to 0.418 (between Decreto Supremo N.° 044-2020-PCM of Peru and Decreto Supremo 4200 of Bolivia). Its mean and standard deviation came to be 0.135 and 0.059, respectively.

Since different studies operationalized multi-dimensions of state capacity with different indicators, I also estimated eight models with indexes and indicators used in other studies. Model 1 used Hanson and Sigman's (2021) Capacity, which represents a latent dimension of state capacity based on 21 indicators of the three dimensions of state capacity. *Difference in capacity* measures the absolute difference in the values of Capacity in 2015 between the two countries of a dyad. Instead of Capacity, Model 2 used the Government Effectiveness indicator of the Worldwide Governance Indicators, which is also used as a single indicator of state capacity (e.g., Serikbayeva et al., 2021). *Difference in government effectiveness* captures the absolute difference in the values of Government Effectiveness in 2019 between the two countries of a dyad. Since Government Effectiveness is also regarded as an indicator of administrative capacity (e.g., Cronert, 2022), I also included indicators of extractive and coercive capacities in Model 3. The former is the total tax revenues as a percentage of GDP, and the latter is logged military expenditures per capita (Hanson & Sigman, 2021). *Difference in tax revenue* and *difference in military expenditure per capita* measure the absolute difference in the values of tax revenues as a percentage of GDP in 2015 and logged military expenditure per capita in 2015 between the two countries of a dyad, respectively.

Model 4 followed Knutsen and Kolvani (2024), who used V-Dem's indicator on impartial administration as a single indicator of state capacity. *Difference in impartial administration* measures the absolute difference in the values of V-Dem's "rigorous and impartial public administration" indicator in 2019 between the two countries of a dyad. Since this indicator is related to administrative capacity, Model 5 included *difference in tax revenue* and *difference in military expenditure per capita* as additional independent variables.

Models 6, 7, and 8 took advantage of various indicators of administrative capacity in addition to *difference in tax revenue* and *difference in military expenditure per capita* which worked to observe the impacts of extractive and coercive capacities. To test delivery, coordination, and analytical capacities mentioned in

González-Bustamante (2021), Model 6 included *difference in government health expenditure per capita*, *difference in division of power index*, and *difference in hospital beds ratio*, respectively.[10] *Difference in government health expenditure per capita* captures the absolute difference in the values of domestic general government health expenditure per capita in US$ in 2019 between the two countries of a dyad, while *difference in division of power index* measures the absolute difference in the values of the division of power index of V-Dem in 2019 between the two countries of a dyad. *Difference in hospital beds ratio* measures the absolute difference in the numbers of hospital beds per 1000 people. Model 7 excluded the *difference in division of power index* following Agostinis and Parthenay (2021),[11] while Model 8 added the *difference in informational capacity,* following Ganga and Schenk (2024), instead of the *difference in division of power index* and *difference in hospital beds ratio.*[12] *Difference in informational capacity* captures the absolute difference in Brambor et al.'s (2020) information capacity index in 2015 between the two countries of a dyad.

Table 6.5 in Appendix summarizes coding and descriptive statistics of these independent variables. In addition, Table 6.6 in Appendix shows coding and descriptive statistics of eight control variables included in the models: *neighboring countries*, *difference in electoral democracy index*, *difference in population density*, *difference in GDP per capita*, *difference in foreign direct investment*, *difference in trade*, *difference in the number of infections*, and *difference in the number of deaths*.

Table 6.2 reports the results of Models 1–8 with standard errors clustered by a dyad. Model 1 verifies Maggetti and Gilardi (2016) that structural equivalence is an indicator related to emulation. The coefficient for *difference in capacity* is negative and significant at the 0.05 level. It suggests that similarity in the general level of state capacity makes two countries issue similar presidential decrees on COVID-19 policies.

My statistical tests revealed that administrative capacity plays a role in emulation of COVID-19 policies. The coefficients for *difference in government health expenditure per capita* are negative and significant in Models 6, 7, and 8, supporting H1a. This finding is consistent with the case between Decreto de Urgencia 026-2020 of Peru and Decreto 3469/2020 of Paraguay, which takes a relatively high value of

---

[10] González-Bustamante (2021) used logged current health expenditure per capita for testing delivery capacity, but here I relied on domestic general government health expenditure per capita for comparing Model 6 with Models 7 and 8. He also used the number of infections and the burden index for analysis capacity, but I used the former for control purpose, while I did not use the latter due to lack of data.

[11] I did not include some variables that were used by Agostinis and Parthenay (2021). For example, I did not include external health expenditure as a percentage of total health expenditure because of its small share in Latin America, nor the number of doctors per 10,000 people and the antiretroviral therapy coverage among people living with HIV due to lack of data.

[12] They also considered the number of military personnel per 1000 people, and the number of police officers per 1000 people as indicators of coercive capacity and, on the other hand, the number of doctors per 1000 people as an indicator of administrative capacity. However, I did not include them due to lack of data.

Table 6.2 Determinants of similarities in presidential decrees

Independent variables	Model 1			Model 2			Model 3			Model 4		
Difference in capacity	−0.034	(0.014)	*									
Difference in government effectiveness				−0.015	(0.014)		−0.016	(0.014)				
Difference in impartial administration										−0.006	(0.006)	
Difference in tax revenue							0.000	(0.001)				
Difference in military expenditure per capita							0.004	(0.002)	*			
Difference in government health expenditure per capita												
Difference in division of power index												
Difference in hospital beds ratio												
Difference in informational capacity												
Neighboring countries	0.002	(0.008)		0.002	(0.008)		0.004	(0.009)		0.000	(0.008)	
Difference in electoral democracy index	0.046	(0.041)		0.037	(0.047)		0.037	(0.046)		0.041	(0.050)	
Difference in population density	−0.000	(0.000)		−0.000	(0.000)		−0.000	(0.000)		0.000	(0.000)	
Difference in GDP per capita	−0.000	(0.000)		−0.000	(0.000)		−0.000	(0.000)		−0.000	(0.000)	
Difference in foreign direct investment	0.000	(0.002)		0.002	(0.002)		0.002	(0.002)		0.000	(0.003)	
Difference in trade	0.000	(0.000)		0.000	(0.000)		−0.000	(0.000)		0.000	(0.000)	
Difference in the number of infections	0.000	(0.000)		−0.000	(0.000)		0.000	(0.000)		−0.000	(0.000)	
Difference in the number of deaths	0.000	(0.000)	*	0.000	(0.000)	*	0.000	(0.000)	*	0.000	(0.000)	*
Constant	0.135	(0.022)	***	0.126	(0.023)	***	0.126	(0.025)	***	0.128	(0.024)	***
R^2	0.073			0.056			0.067			0.055		
N	10,733			10,733			10,733			10,733		

*Independent variables for testing the impacts of state capacity are in bold. Robust standard errors in parentheses. *p < 0.05: **p < 0.01; ***p < 0.001*

Table 6.2 (continued)

Independent variables	Model 5			Model 6			Model 7			Model 8		
Difference in capacity												
Difference in government effectiveness												
Difference in impartial administration	−0.009	(0.006)										
Difference in tax revenue	0.000	(0.001)		−0.001	(0.001)		−0.001	(0.001)		0.000	(0.001)	
Difference in military expenditure per capita	0.005	(0.002)	*	0.007	(0.003)	*	0.005	(0.002)	**	0.007	(0.002)	**
Difference in government health expenditure per capita				−0.000	(0.000)	**	−0.000	(0.000)	*	−0.000	(0.000)	**
Difference in division of power index				−0.031	(0.018)							
Difference in hospital beds ratio				0.007	(0.007)		0.008	(0.007)				
Difference in informational capacity										0.090	(0.061)	
Neighboring countries	0.002	(0.009)		0.009	(0.009)		0.008	(0.009)		0.007	(0.008)	
Difference in electoral democracy index	0.055	(0.048)		0.011	(0.044)		0.020	(0.044)		−0.024	(0.058)	
Difference in population density	−0.000	(0.000)		−0.000	(0.000)		−0.000	(0.000)		−0.000	(0.000)	
Difference in GDP per capita	−0.000	(0.000)		0.000	(0.000)	*	0.000	(0.000)		0.000	(0.000)	*
Difference in foreign direct investment	−0.000	(0.003)		0.000	(0.002)		0.000	(0.002)		0.000	(0.004)	
Difference in trade	−0.000	(0.000)		−0.000	(0.000)		−0.000	(0.000)		−0.000	(0.000)	
Difference in the number of infections	−0.000	(0.000)		−0.000	(0.000)		−0.000	(0.000)		−0.000	(0.000)	
Difference in the number of deaths	0.000	(0.000)	*	0.000	(0.000)		0.000	(0.000)		0.000	(0.000)	*
Constant	0.129	(0.026)	***	0.143	(0.025)	***	0.141	(0.025)	***	0.126	(0.032)	***
R^2	0.068			0.089			0.085			0.094		
N	10,733			10,733			10,733			9676		

Independent variables for testing the impacts of state capacity are in bold. Robust standard errors in parentheses. $^{*}p < 0.05$: $^{**}p < 0.01$; $^{***}p < 0.001$

0.385 in *cosine* and a relatively low value of 40 in *difference in government health expenditure per capita*. The former decree introduced various measures against COVID-19 on March 15, 2020, and the latter decree authorized the Ministry of Finance to finance relevant state organizations and entities on March 18, 2020. It is possible that the Paraguayan government took advantage of some parts of the Peruvian decree, considering that their levels of government health expenditure were similar.

The other variables on administrative capacity do not generate significant coefficients in Models 2–8. Neither *difference in government effectiveness* nor *difference in administration* generates significant coefficients as an indicator of general state capacity as well as that of administrative capacity. In Model 6, the coefficient for *difference in division of power index*, which captures coordination capacity, is negative but not statistically significant. *Difference in hospital beds ratio* in Models 6 and 7, which captures analysis capacity, and *difference in informational capacity* in Model 8 also do not generate significant coefficients. As argued in the introductory chapter of this book, a country with high state capacity in some issue areas does not necessarily hold the same level of state capacity in other issue areas. This statistical test shows that the emulation of COVID-19 policies in Latin America at the very early stage of the pandemic was related to delivery capacity in health issue areas.

What about coercive capacity in the emulation of policies during the pandemic? This statistical test does not support H1b. In all the models that include the *difference in military expenditure per capita* variable, positive and significant coefficients are generated, which contradicts H1b. However, this result should be interpreted with caution, since this variable has a value of 0 for Costa Rica and Panama. Costa Rica abolished its military in 1948, while Panama abandoned it in 1990 after the US invasion in 1989 that overthrew Manuel Noriega's dictatorship. It is thus possible that Costa Rica and Panama make the variance of this variable excessively large. The correlation coefficient for *difference in military expenditure per capita* is 0.041 and statistically significant in my dataset, but it changes to negative (−0.035) and significant at the 0.01 level if we exclude Costa Rica and Panama.

Most of the control variables do not generate significant coefficients except for *difference in the number of deaths* in Models 1–5 and 8, and *difference in GDP per capita* in Models 6 and 8.

6.6 Testing H2

The statistical tests conducted in the previous section support H1a with regard to the role of administrative capacity in the emulation process and reject H1b with regard to the role of coercive capacity. Which countries are more likely to be senders and receivers of emulations of COVID-19 policies? To test H1, I included a series of independent variables that capture the absolute differences in the levels of various dimensions of state capacity between the two countries of a dyad. I considered the individual values of the variables for each country in exchange for taking the absolute difference to test H2.

The models for testing H2 used *capacity*, *government effectiveness*, *impartial administration*, *tax revenue*, *military expenditure per capita*, *government health expenditure per capita*, *division of power index*, *hospital beds ratio*, and *information capacity*. I used the issue dates of presidential decrees to identify senders and receivers and regarded a country in a dyad as a sender if it issued the decree in question earlier than the other country (a receiver). I then generated these independent variables for senders and receivers and included the pair of the variables in the same equations. Table 6.7 in Appendix summarizes coding and descriptive statistics of these independent variables.

Table 6.3 shows the results for Models 1I-8I with standard errors clustered by a dyad. All the models included the same control variables as Models 1–8. Overall, the results of this statistical test support H2b regarding the receivers' administrative capacity characteristics. *Government health expenditure per capita (receiver)* generates negative and significant coefficients in Models 6I-8I. Furthermore, the coefficients for *government effectiveness (receiver)* in Models 2I and 3I, as well as *impartial administration (receiver)* in Model 5I, are also negative and significant. These results imply that not only the countries with lower delivery capacity in public health but also those with lower general administration capacity tend to imitate the policies of other countries, even though the *hospital beds ratio (receiver)* generates a positive and significant coefficient in Model 7I. Model 1I also shows that a country with a lower level of general state capacity is more likely to emulate decrees issued in other countries.

Regarding the characteristics of the senders, my statistical tests show mixed but interesting results. On the one hand, the coefficients for *hospital beds ratio (sender)* in Models 6I and 7I as well as for *information capacity (sender)* in Model 8I are positive and significant. Given that González-Bustamante (2021) considered hospital beds ratio an indicator of analysis capacity, these results indicate that countries tend to imitate policies of a country with a higher level of analysis and information capacity, which supports H2a.

On the other hand, *government health expenditure per capita (sender)*, another indicator of administrative capacity, produces negative and significant coefficients in Models 6I-8I, which contradicts H2a. In addition, *government effectiveness (sender)* in Models 2I and 3I and *impartial administration (sender)* in Model 5I also generate negative and significant coefficients. How can these findings be understood?

Considering state capacity weakness may help us generate a possible interpretation of the findings. As predicted in H2a, it is true that COVID-19 policies adopted in other countries with a higher analysis and information capacity were attractive to policymakers because their qualities were guaranteed even if nobody knew their consequences. However, given the urgency as well as weak state capacity, many policymakers had to make realistic decisions within a very limited time period. Consequently, it is possible that they tended to imitate policies of other countries with a *lower* level of administrative capacity since such policies should be easy to implement with limited state capacity. The negative and significant coefficients for *government effectiveness (sender)* in Models 2I and 3I, *military expenditure per capita (sender)* in Models 3I and 5I-8I, and *tax revenue (sender)* in Model 8I might fit such an interpretation, but more research on this issue is necessary.

Table 6.3 Determinants of similarities in presidential decrees (with individual state capacity variables)

Independent variables	Model 1I			Model 2I			Model 3I			Model 4I		
Capacity (sender)	−0.011	(0.008)										
Capacity (receiver)	−0.034	(0.007)	***									
Government effectiveness (sender)				−0.018	(0.006)	**	−0.022	(0.005)	***			
Government effectiveness (receiver)				−0.025	(0.007)	**	−0.028	(0.005)	***			
Impartial administration (sender)										−0.002	(0.003)	
Impartial administration (receiver)										−0.004	(0.004)	
Tax revenue (sender)							−0.001	(0.001)				
Tax revenue (receiver)							0.000	(0.001)				
Military expenditure per capita (sender)							−0.006	(0.001)	***			
Military expenditure per capita (receiver)							−0.010	(0.001)	***			
Government health expenditure per capita (sender)												
Government health expenditure per capita (receiver)												
Division of power index (sender)												
Division of power index (receiver)												
Hospital beds ratio (sender)												
Hospital beds ratio (receiver)												
Information capacity (sender)												
Information capacity (receiver)												
(control variables)												
Constant	0.164	(0.030)	***	0.136	(0.021)	***	0.226	(0.038)	***	0.136	(0.030)	***
R^2	0.081			0.089			0.158			0.056		
N	10,733			10,733			10,733			10,733		

Each model includes the same control variables as its original model in Table 6.2
Robust standard errors in parentheses
$*p < 0.05$; $**p < 0.01$; $***p < 0.001$

Table 6.3 Continued

Independent variables	Model 5I			Model 6I			Model 7I			Model 8I		
Capacity (sender)												
Capacity (receiver)												
Government effectiveness (sender)												
Government effectiveness (receiver)												
Impartial administration (sender)	–0.007	(0.003)	**									
Impartial administration (receiver)	–0.010	(0.002)	***									
Tax revenue (sender)	–0.001	(0.001)		–0.001	(0.001)		–0.001	(0.001)		–0.002	(0.001)	**
Tax revenue (receiver)	0.000	(0.001)		0.001	(0.001)		0.000	(0.001)		–0.001	(0.001)	
Military expenditure per capita (sender)	–0.006	(0.001)	***	–0.007	(0.001)	***	–0.008	(0.002)	***	–0.004	(0.001)	**
Military expenditure per capita (receiver)	–0.011	(0.002)	***	–0.013	(0.002)	***	–0.012	(0.002)	***	–0.008	(0.001)	***
Government health expenditure per capita (sender)				–0.000	(0.000)	***	–0.000	(0.000)	**	–0.000	(0.000)	***
Government health expenditure per capita (receiver)				–0.000	(0.000)	***	–0.000	(0.000)	***	–0.000	(0.000)	***
Division of power index (sender)				–0.019	(0.012)							
Division of power index (receiver)				0.009	(0.016)							
Hospital beds ratio (sender)				0.012	(0.005)	*	0.011	(0.005)	*			
Hospital beds ratio (receiver)				0.011	(0.006)		0.012	(0.006)	*			
Information capacity (sender)										0.217	(0.046)	***
Information capacity (receiver)										0.064	(0.047)	
(control variables)												
Constant	0.256	(0.051)	***	0.250	(0.030)	***	0.244	(0.029)	***	0.087	(0.057)	
R^2	0.136			0.159			0.158			0.187		
N	10,733			10,733			10,733			9676		

Each model includes the same control variables as its original model in Table 6.2
Robust standard errors in parentheses
*$p < 0.05$: **$p < 0.01$; ***$p < 0.001$

6.7 Conclusion

Did state capacity play a crucial role in the diffusion of non-pharmaceutical interventions in Latin America? If so, which dimension of state capacity did matter? I studied these questions combining a dyadic approach with a text analysis of presidential decrees issued in 12 countries between February and March 2020. Focusing on the very first state of the pandemic allowed me to isolate emulation from other mechanisms of policy diffusion because policymakers were forced to make decisions without knowing the consequences of policies of other countries. To answer the research questions, I first reviewed social science literature on the role of state capacity in the case of COVID-19 and identified indicators that capture extractive, coercive, and administrative dimensions of state capacity. Combining it with the literature on policy diffusion that identified emulation, learning, and competition as its mechanisms, I hypothesized that a similar level of administrative and coercive capacities makes two countries issue similar presidential decrees. I also hypothesized that presidential decrees issued by a country with a higher administrative capacity tend to be copied by others, and that a country with a lower administrative capacity tends to emulate presidential decrees issued by other countries.

Statistical tests with the dependent variable generated via text analysis and independent variables that capture various dimensions of state capacity revealed that the emulation of COVID-19 policies in Latin America at the very early stage of the pandemic was related to delivery capacity in public health issues. Moreover, countries with a lower general administrative capacity or a lower delivery capacity in public health tended to imitate the presidential decrees of other countries.

This chapter demonstrated the important role of state capacity in the process of COVID-19 policy diffusion in Latin America. However, some questions remain unanswered. First, we expect to conduct another analysis with more cases, since this study only focused on 12 out of 20 Latin American countries due to lack of data. Second, it is expected to conduct additional studies to interpret the mixed results on the characteristics of senders in the process of policy diffusion, since the statistical analysis of this chapter showed that a country with a higher level of analysis and information capacity tended to be imitated, but that a country with a lower administrative and coercive capacity also had a similar tendency. My tentative interpretation rests on the assumption that policymakers were forced to make a realistic decision to implement easier policies with limited state capacity, but it should be verified by other analyses in the future.

Acknowledgments I would like to appreciate all the comments on an earlier version of this chapter at the International Workshop "Comparative Perspectives on State Capacity and the COVID-19 Pandemic in Latin America" at El Colegio de México on March 22, 2024. This study was supported by JSPS KAKENHI No. 20KK0024.

Appendix

Table 6.4 Sources of presidential decrees used for this study

Country	Source and URL
Mexico	Diario Oficial de la Federación https://www.dof.gob.mx/
Guatemala	Secretaría General de la Presidencia https://sgp.gob.gt/web/index.php/servicios/decretos-gub-disposiciones-pre
Costa Rica	Sistema Costarricense de Información Jurídica https://pgrweb.go.cr/scij/avanzada_pgr.aspx
Panama	Gaceta Oficial https://www.gacetaoficial.gob.pa/
Dominican Republic	Consultoría Jurídica del Poder Ejecutivo https://www.consultoria.gov.do/consulta/
Colombia	Sistema Único de Información Normativa https://www.suin-juriscol.gov.co/legislacion/normatividad.html
Peru	Plataforma Digital Única del Estado Peruano https://www.gob.pe/busquedas
Bolivia	Gaceta Oficial de Bolivia http://www.gacetaoficialdebolivia.gob.bo/normas/
Chile	Ley Chile, Biblioteca del Congreso Nacional https://www.bcn.cl/leychile/
Paraguay	Portal de Normas y Decretos, Presidencia de la República de Paraguay https://decretos.presidencia.gov.py/#/home
Argentina	Boletín Oficial de la República Argentina https://www.boletinoficial.gob.ar/
Uruguay	Normativa, Presidencia de la República https://www.gub.uy/presidencia/institucional/normativa

All the URLs were accessed on January 31, 2025

Table 6.5 Coding and descriptive statistics of independent variables for testing H1

Independent variable	Coding	Min.	Max.	Mean	S.D.
Difference in capacity	The absolute difference between the two countries of a dyad in terms of Hanson and Sigman's (2021) Capacity in 2015	0.019	1.381	0.403	0.298
Difference in government effectiveness	The absolute difference between the two countries of a dyad in terms of the Government Effectiveness indicator of the Worldwide Governance Indicators in 2019	0.010	1.650	0.520	0.356
Difference in tax revenue	The absolute difference between the two countries of a dyad in terms of tax revenues as a percentage of GDP in 2015	0.010	14.000	5.640	3.333

(continued)

Table 6.5 (continued)

Independent variable	Coding	Min.	Max.	Mean	S.D.
Difference in military expenditure per capita	The absolute difference between the two countries of a dyad in terms of logged military expenditure per capita in 2015	0.000	5.653	1.809	1.823
Difference in impartial administration	The absolute difference between the two countries of a dyad in terms of V-Dem's "rigorous and impartial public administration" indicator in 2019	0.043	3.779	1.136	0.879
Difference in government health expenditure per capita	The absolute difference between the two countries of a dyad in terms of domestic general government health expenditure per capita in US$ in 2019	17.000	1020.000	341.233	243.572
Difference in division of power index	The absolute difference between the two countries of a dyad in terms of V-Dem's division of power index in 2019	0.000	0.520	0.176	0.201
Difference in hospital beds ratio	The absolute difference between the two countries of a dyad in terms of the numbers of hospital beds per 1000 people in 2019	0.010	3.200	1.017	0.810
Difference in informational capacity	The absolute difference between the two countries of a dyad in terms of Brambor et al.'s (2020) information capacity index in 2015	0.000	0.217	0.077	0.050

Sources: The data on *difference in capacity*, *difference in military expenditure per capita*, and *difference in informational capacity* were obtained from Hanson and Sigman (2021), while those on *difference in impartial administration* and *difference in division of power index* were obtained from V-Dem (https://www.v-dem.net/data/the-v-dem-dataset/). World Bank's Worldwide Governance Indicators (https://www.worldbank.org/en/publication/worldwide-governance-indicators) and World Development Indicators (https://datatopics.worldbank.org/world-development-indicators/) were used to generate *difference in government effectiveness* and *difference in tax revenue*. *Difference in government health expenditure per capita* and *difference in hospital beds ratio* were based on Global Health Expenditure Database, WHO (https://apps.who.int/nha/database/ViewData/Indicators/en) and PAHO (https://opendata.paho.org/en/core-indicators/core-indicators-dashboard), respectively. All the websites of the sources were accessed on January 31, 2025

Table 6.6 Coding and descriptive statistics of control variables

Control variable	Coding	Min.	Max.	Mean	S.D.
Neighboring countries	1 = A dyad contained presidential decrees of the countries that border each other, 0 = otherwise	0.000	1.000	0.248	0.432
Difference in electoral democracy index	The absolute difference in the values of the electoral democracy index of V-Dem in 2019 between the two countries of a dyad	0.010	0.420	0.160	0.096
Difference in population density	The absolute difference between the two countries of a dyad in terms of the number of people per square kilometers of land area in 2019	0.030	215.260	43.386	50.088
Difference in GDP per capita	The absolute difference between the two countries of a dyad in terms of GDP per capita (constant 2015 US$) in 2019	171.250	14486.060	5325.289	3715.048
Difference in foreign direct investment	The absolute difference between the two countries of a dyad in terms of the net inflows of foreign direct investment as percentage of GDP in 2019	0.030	6.540	2.172	1.372
Difference in trade	The absolute difference between the two countries of a dyad in terms of trade to GDP ratio in 2019	1.210	47.800	18.127	11.502
Difference in the number of infections	The absolute difference between the two countries of a dyad in terms of the number of COVID infections as of March 31, 2020	11.000	2061.000	611.949	440.873
Difference in the number of deaths	The absolute difference between the two countries of a dyad in terms of the number of COVID deaths as of March 29, 2020	0.000	71.000	32.041	29.831

Sources: The data on *neighboring countries* and *difference in electoral democracy index* were obtained from Nation Master (https://www.nationmaster.com/country-info/stats/Background/Neighboring-countries-and-territories#google_vignette) and V-Dem (https://www.v-dem.net/data/the-v-dem-dataset/), respectively. *Difference in the number of infections* and *difference in the number of deaths* are based on WHO (https://data.who.int/dashboards/covid19/), while the other variables are based on World Development Indicators, World Bank (https://datatopics.worldbank.org/world-development-indicators/). All the websites of the sources were accessed on January 31, 2025

Table 6.7 Coding and descriptive statistics of independent variables for testing H2

Independent variable	Coding	Min.	Max.	Mean	S.D.
Capacity	Hanson and Sigman's (2021) Capacity in 2015	0.122	1.503	0.695	0.346
				0.748	0.334
Government effectiveness	The Government Effectiveness indicator of the Worldwide Governance Indicators in 2019	−0.790	0.860	−0.048	0.443
				−0.013	0.416
Tax revenue	Tax revenues as a percentage of GDP in 2015	9.700	23.700	16.000	4.355
				15.488	4.220
Military expenditure per capita	Logged military expenditure per capita in 2015	0.000	5.653	4.027	1.835
				4.324	1.610
Impartial administration	V-Dem's "rigorous and impartial public administration" indicator in 2019	−0.857	2.922	0.833	0.972
				0.955	0.978
Government health expenditure per capita	Domestic general government health expenditure per capita in US$ in 2019	107.000	1127.000	449.420	279.263
				488.130	285.523
Division of power index	V-Dem's division of power index in 2019	0.460	0.990	0.833	0.209
				0.841	0.206
Hospital beds ratio	The numbers of hospital beds per 1000 people in 2019	0.500	3.700	1.707	0.749
				1.975	0.947
Informational capacity	Brambor et al.'s (2020) information capacity index in 2015	0.577	0.794	0.697	0.064
				0.704	0.059

The values of mean and standard deviation in the upper and lower rows of each variable are those for senders and receivers, respectively. Sources for these variables are same as the sources for generating variables for testing H1, which is summarized in Table 6.5

References

Agostinis, G., & Parthenay, K. (2021). Exploring the determinants of regional health governance modes in the global south: A comparative analysis of central and South America. *Review of International Studies, 47*(4), 399–421.

Borgatti, S. P., & Grosser, T. J. (2015). Structural equivalence: Meaning and measures. In J. D. Wright (Ed.), *International encyclopedia of the social & behavioral sciences* (2nd ed., pp. 621–625). Elsevier.

Brambor, T., Goenaga, A., Lindvall, J., & Teorell, J. (2020). The lay of the land: Information capacity and the modern state. *Comparative Political Studies, 53*(2), 175–213.

Cameron, M. A., Hurtado, V., Sosa Villagarcia, P., & Gombata, M. (2023). A tale of two crashes: Pandemic politics in Brazil and Peru. *Latin American Perspectives, 50*(4), 248–267.

Centeno, M. A., Kohli, A., & Yashar, D. J. (2017). Unpacking states in the developing world: Capacity, performance, and politics. In M. A. Centeno, A. Kohli, & D. J. Yashar (Eds.), *States in the developing world* (pp. 1–32). Cambridge University Press.

Cingolani, L. (2013). The state of state capacity: A review of concepts, evidence, and measures. *MERIT Working Papers 2013-053*, United Nations University-MERIT.

Coppedge, M., Gerring, J., Knutsen, C. H., Lindberg, S. I., Teorell, J., Altman, D., Angiolillo, F., Bernhard, M., Borella, C., Cornell, A., Fish, M. S., Fox, L., Gastaldi, L., Gjerløw, H., Glynn, A., Good God, A., Grahn, S., Hicken, A., Kinzelbach, K., Marquardt, K. L., McMann, K., Mechkova, V., Neundorf, A., Paxton, P., Pemstein, D., Rydén, O., von Römer, J., Seim, B., Sigman, R., Skaaning, S.-E., Staton, J., Sundström, A., Tzelgov, E., Uberti, L., Wang, Y.-T., Wig, T., & Ziblatt, D. (2024). V-Dem codebook v14. *Varieties of Democracy (V-Dem) Project.*

Croissant, A., & Hellmann, O. (2023). Introduction: Democracy and state capacity during times of crisis. In *Democracy, state capacity, and the governance of COVID-19 in Asia-Oceania* (pp. 1–21). Routledge.

Cronert, A. (2022). Precaution and proportionality in pandemic politics: Democracy, state capacity, and COVID-19-related school closures around the world. *Journal of Public Policy, 42*(4), 705–729.

Düpont, N., & Rachuj, M. (2022). The ties that bind: Text similarities and conditional diffusion among parties. *British Journal of Political Science, 52*(2), 613–630.

Flores-Macías, G. A. (2022). *Contemporary state building: Elite taxation and public safety in Latin America.* Cambridge University Press.

Ganga, P. D., & Schenk, C. (2024). State capacity during crisis: Exploring varieties of state capacity in the COVID-19 pandemic. *Territory, Politics, Governance*, 1–22.

González-Bustamante, B. (2021). Evolution and early government responses to COVID-19 in South America. *World Development, 137*, 105180.

Han, J., Kamber, M., & Pei, J. (2012). *Data mining: Concepts and techniques* (3rd ed.). Morgan Kaufmann.

Hanson, J. K., & Sigman, R. (2021). Leviathan's latent dimensions: Measuring state capacity for comparative political research. *The Journal of Politics, 83*(4), 1495–1510.

Hinkle, R. K. (2015). Into the words: Using statutory text to explore the impact of federal courts on state policy diffusion. *American Journal of Political Science, 59*(4), 1002–1021.

Huang, A. (2008). Similarity measures for text document clustering. Proceedings of the sixth New Zealand computer science research student conference (NZCSRSC 2008), Christchurch, New Zealand.

Knutsen, C. H., & Kolvani, P. (2024). Fighting the disease or manipulating the data? Democracy, state capacity, and the COVID-19 pandemic. *World Politics, 76*(3), 543–593.

Kurtz, M. J. (2013). *Latin American state building in comparative perspective: Social foundations of institutional order*. Cambridge University Press.

Leonisio, R., & Strijbis, O. (2012). El problema de la traducción en el análisis cuantitativo de textos. Aplicación de Wordscores y Wordfish a las mociones de censura contra el lehendakari Ibarretxe. *Revista Española de Ciencia Política, 30*, 111–120.

Lesch, M., & Millar, H. (2022). Crisis, uncertainty and urgency: Processes of learning and emulation in tax policy making. *West European Politics, 45*(4), 930–952.
Lundgren, M., Klamberg, M., Sundström, K., & Dahlqvist, J. (2020). Emergency powers in response to COVID-19: Policy diffusion, democracy, and preparedness. *Nordic Journal of Human Rights, 38*(4), 305–318.
Mann, M. (1993). *The sources of social power, volume II: The rise of classes and nation-states, 1760–1914*. Cambridge University Press.
Maggetti, M., & Gilardi, F. (2016). Problems (and solutions) in the measurement of policy diffusion mechanisms. *Journal of Public Policy, 36*(1), 87–107.
Sebhatu, A., Wennberg, K., Arora-Jonsson, S., & Lindberg, S. I. (2020). Explaining the homogeneous diffusion of COVID-19 nonpharmaceutical interventions across heterogeneous countries. *Proceedings of the National Academy of Sciences, 117*(35), 21201–21208.
Serikbayeva, B., Abdulla, K., & Oskenbayev, Y. (2021). State capacity in responding to COVID-19. *International Journal of Public Administration, 44*(11–12), 920–930.
Shipan, C. R., & Volden, C. (2008). The mechanisms of policy diffusion. *American Journal of Political Science, 52*(4), 840–857.
Tosun, J. (2023). Policy responses to the COVID-19 pandemic: An aggregate-level comparative analysis. In A. Croissant & O. Hellmann (Eds.), *Democracy, state capacity, and the governance of COVID-19 in Asia-Oceania* (pp. 22–42). Routledge.
Weber, M. (1978). *Economy and society: An outline of interpretive sociology*. University of California Press.
Yen, W.-T., Liu, L.-Y., Won, E., & Testriono. (2022). The imperative of state capacity in public health crisis: Asia's early COVID-19 policy responses. *Governance, 35*(3), 777–798.
Yi, H., & Liu, I. (2022). Executive leadership, policy tourism, and policy diffusion among local governments. *Public Administration Review, 82*(6), 1024–1041.
Zhang, Y., & Zhu, X. (2019). Multiple mechanisms of policy diffusion in China. *Public Management Review, 21*(4), 495–514.

Chapter 7
Collaborative Governance as a Policy Strategy to Combat the Covid-19 Pandemic: Lessons from Latin America

Matías Bianchi, Florencia Coda, and Sofía Santamarina

7.1 Introduction

In recent years, there has been a growing academic interest in understanding policy responses to wicked problems: challenges characterized by their multidimensional complexity, interconnected nature, and the uncertainty surrounding their origins and potential solutions (Rittel & Webber, 1973; Emerson & Nabatchi, 2015). These problems require innovative governance models that transcend traditional government boundaries—given their dynamic nature and the interdependence of their dimensions. Phenomena such as climate change, forced migrations, illicit trafficking, and global pandemics transcend national and sectoral borders, demanding governance approaches integrating diverse actors in coordinated and effective responses.

In this context, the Covid-19 outbreak highlighted the urgency of rethinking governance models in the face of problems that do not recognize sectoral or geographic boundaries. Although initially perceived as a health crisis, its impacts quickly spread to the economic, social, and political realms. In Latin America, this crisis exposed the structural limitations of states in articulating comprehensive responses. The region, which represents 8% of the world's population but accounted for nearly 30% of Covid-19 deaths (CEPAL, 2021), faced significant challenges due to its high levels of inequality, labor and economic informality, and institutional fragmentation.

This chapter seeks to understand the complexity of the policy responses to the pandemic in that region. Particularly, it aims to unpack the collaborative governance (CG) schemes that were implemented in specific counties. CG is a policy approach

M. Bianchi (✉) · S. Santamarina
Asuntos del Sur, Ciudad Autónoma de Buenos Aires, Argentina
e-mail: matias.bianchi@asuntosdelsur.org

F. Coda
Universidad Torcuato Di Tella, Autónoma de Buenos Aires, Argentina
e-mail: fcoda@utdt.edu

I. Okada (ed.), *COVID-19 and State Capacity in Latin America*, Latin American Societies, https://doi.org/10.1007/978-3-032-15572-6_7

that seeks to replace traditional approaches to policy formulation and implementation (Ansell & Gash, 2008). CG transcends traditional hierarchical structures by promoting the participation of diverse actors in addressing problems, recognizing their interdependence and complexity, and proposing interdisciplinary and intersectoral solutions.

This approach, led by studies of policies in the United States and Europe (see Emerson & Tina, 2015), emphasizes that challenges of the magnitude of the pandemic require robust state capacities, as well as joint efforts with other sectors and levels of government. However, the experience of Latin America shows that in contexts of weak political institutions, lack of resources, and political instability, it is difficult to see CG emerge from a formalized process like in the Global North. Yet, CG does occur. It did play a crucial role in facilitating coordination between diverse actors and implementing policy solutions with positive impacts. It emerges as a compensatory mechanism, most of the time in an *Ad Hoc* manner, replacing or supporting weak institutional arrangements. Therefore, this chapter shows that CG presents particular characteristics in countries of the Global South distinct from those of the Global North, which affect the dynamics of collaboration and, therefore, it proposes a contribution to the literature of institutional capabilities, and particularly to CG.

The research brings specific cases from six different countries in Latin America that show different arrangement, particularly focusing on vulnerable contexts: ethnic youth in Guatemala and Colombia (Afro-youth from the Pacific region), women in the informal sector in Mexico and Bolivia (El Alto and La Paz), migrants in transit in Mexico, as well as marginalized urban communities in Argentina (in the municipalities of San Martín, Tres de Febrero, Quilmes, and Avellaneda in Buenos Aires province) and Chile (the periphery of Santiago: La Pintana, Cerro Navia, and Renca). These populations faced unique challenges such as labor precariousness, unequal access to healthcare services, and structural discrimination, which conditioned the collaborative dynamics. The data used here comes from "COLABORA. Lat: Toward a New Post-COVID-19 Governance Model," a project developed between 2020 and 2024 (Colabora.Lat 2022).[1] The cases are built from statistical data, in-depth interviews, focus groups, and secondary sources. The concepts and cases are developed at length in Cyr et al. (2025).

This chapter first revisits conceptual approaches to CG and its connection to the literature of institutional capabilities. It particularly develops the experience of Ad Hoc arrangements that have limited participation of national governments. It highlights the importance to contextualize those arrangements to the power dynamics and the diversity of actors present in the territory. Based on the empirical experience

[1] COLABORA.Lat had an Implementation Council formed by the organization Asuntos del Sur from Argentina, the National University of San Martín from Argentina, the Faculty of Humanities of the University of Santiago de Chile, the Friedrich Ebert Foundation in Bolivia, the organization Diálogos from Guatemala, the organization Nosotrxs from Mexico, and the ICESI University from Colombia. It was supported by the International Development Research Centre (IDRC) of the Canadian government https://colabora.lat/

of Latin America, this chapter makes a substantive contribution on how CG operates in countries of the Global South with weaker institutions and large power asymmetries.

7.2 Conceptual Approaches to Collaborative Governance

In recent decades, a new governance dynamic has emerged that seeks to replace traditional approaches to policy formulation and implementation: CG (Ansell & Gash, 2008). This model is characterized by a partnership approach oriented toward consensus, developed through formal deliberation between public agencies and non-state stakeholders (Barandiarán et al., 2022). CG transcends traditional hierarchical structures by promoting the participation of diverse actors in addressing problems, recognizing their interdependence and complexity, and proposing interdisciplinary and intersectoral solutions. In this sense, in contrast to the traditional approach, CG advocates for broadening the approach to social problems, particularly in complex or changing contexts.

Initially studied in the United States and Europe (Emerson & Tina, 2015), the concept emerged as a response to the need for a flexible and adaptable approach to public management that would allow contemporary challenges to be addressed more effectively. In this way, CG is defined as a process in which public state agencies share power with non-state actors in formulating and implementing public policies or programs (Ulibarri et al., 2023; Bianchi et al., 2021). This process, initiated by public institutions, formally incorporates the direct participation of non-state actors in decision-making. Following Cyr et al. (2021), CG can be understood as a series of instances/meetings of exchange between organizations, groups, and/or different institutions aimed at designing and implementing a policy or action. In these instances, all actors involved in the exchange maintain their own identity, are free from external coercion, and engage in exchanges on equal terms. This collective decision-making process seeks to bring together knowledge and experiences from different stakeholders (Bryson et al., 2006, p. 44) to design more effective policies (Ansell & Gash, 2008).

A central feature of CG is the active participation of diverse actors oriented toward consensus in decision-making through negotiation among participants, as opposed to imposing a solution by a central authority. Furthermore, its functioning involves a process of deliberation and dialogue centered on formal institutions, where trust between actors is crucial for collaboration success (Barandiarán et al., 2022).

However, in a region like Latin America, where institutions are weak and political instability is pronounced (Vian, 2008), it is difficult to see CG emerge from formalized processes. The region is characterized by shifting political actors, instability that prevents the development of behavioral norms, and a lack of trust, all of which become obstacles to any form of cooperation (Bennett et al., 2018). Beyond the problems associated with government institutions, actors in the Global South tend to have fewer resources. These "lower resource environments" (Bennett et al., 2018) hinder the institutionalization of collaboration because they make long-term investment uncertain. Additionally, there are de facto powers—such as oligarchic elites or organized crime—operating outside of the formal state, obstructing the development of relationships between the state and society.

These challenges raise doubts about the direct applicability of existing CG theories in Global South contexts, as they were largely developed based on experiences from the Global North. However, during the Covid-19 pandemic, CG played a crucial role in facilitating coordination among diverse actors and implementing innovative policies with greater efficiency, impact, and legitimacy. This suggests that while the conceptual foundations of CG do not fully align with the realities of the Global South, it does apply *de facto*. CG just takes on specific forms in these contexts. This chapter analyzes these particular characteristics and how they manifested during the pandemic.

Understanding the characteristics of CG in Latin America requires first analyzing its relationship with state capacities. The effectiveness and reach of CG largely depend on the state's ability to engage with non-state actors, mobilize resources, and build trust in contexts marked by structural inequalities.

7.3 Collaborative Governance and State Capacities in Latin America

The literature on CG emphasizes the central role of the state in fostering and sustaining collaboration with other actors. A strong and capable state provides the necessary institutional framework, resources, and legitimacy to facilitate multi-actor partnerships, ensuring their continuity and effectiveness (Ansell & Gash, 2008; Emerson & Tina, 2015). In high-capacity states, governments act as coordinators and enablers of CG, establishing stable mechanisms that integrate civil society, private actors, and local governments into decision-making processes. These collaborations are often institutionalized, supported by regulatory frameworks, and embedded in long-term governance strategies.

The state is widely recognized as a central actor in governance, as there are certain functions that only it can perform both legitimately and effectively. The interactive governance paradigm (Torfing et al., 2012) highlights key governance activities that non-state actors are not equipped to carry out, such as articulating shared priorities, balancing competing interests, delivering services tied to fundamental rights, and ensuring accountability. From this perspective, collaborative models that exclude the state appear limited in their capacity to address these crucial functions, making the state's involvement indispensable.

However, in Latin America, state capacity tends to be weaker, limiting the government's ability to assume this enabling role. Rather than serving as a structured governance regime, CG in the region often emerges as a compensatory mechanism, filling gaps left by under-resourced or absent state institutions. Instead of fostering collaboration proactively, governments frequently rely on CG as an emergency response strategy, delegating responsibilities to civil society and the private sector to address urgent policy challenges. This reactive and fragmented approach prevents CG from becoming a long-term governance tool and instead leads to short-lived, dynamic arrangements.

Yet, while state capacity remains generally low across the region, it is not uniform. The degree of institutional strength varies among countries, shaping how CG emerges and functions in different contexts. Chile and Argentina demonstrate more consolidated state structures, with stronger bureaucratic institutions and service delivery systems. However, Argentina faces significant intergovernmental coordination challenges, which hinder policy implementation effectiveness (Rodríguez & Ortiz, 2021). In contrast, Bolivia and Guatemala struggle with pronounced institutional weaknesses. Bolivia's administrative limitations prevent the effective implementation of inclusive policies, particularly in resource-limited settings (World Bank, 2024). Similarly, Guatemala's weak institutions and lack of robust information systems undermine the state's ability to address critical needs (UNESCO, 2020).

Colombia and Mexico occupy an intermediate position. Colombia has made strides in designing inclusive policies but continues to face stark regional disparities, particularly in rural and conflict-affected areas (UNESCO, 2020). Mexico presents a mixed scenario, where governance structures vary widely across states, reflecting both strong local initiatives and federal-level governance challenges.

These variations in state capacity directly shape the characteristics of CG in each country. Where the state has more institutional strength, collaborative arrangements tend to have more structure, greater continuity, and stronger government engagement. Conversely, in low-capacity environments, CG is more likely to emerge in an ad hoc and informal manner, with civil society taking the lead in policy implementation.

The relationship between state capacity and CG is therefore crucial to understanding how collaboration unfolds in Latin America. In contexts of high state capacity, CG can be an effective governance tool, where the government actively coordinates partnerships, mobilizes resources, and institutionalizes collaboration over time. In contrast, in low-capacity environments, CG becomes a necessity rather than a strategic choice, compensating for governance deficits rather than complementing state action.

The Covid-19 pandemic provided a critical test of this relationship. The crisis required rapid, coordinated responses across multiple sectors and levels of government, exposing both the strengths and weaknesses of existing governance structures. In low-capacity states, governments struggled to respond effectively, leading to greater reliance on non-state actors to manage service delivery and crisis response. This dynamic reinforced CG's role as an emergency governance tool, but also highlighted its limitations: without state support, many collaborative arrangements remained short-term and lacked the resources or institutional backing to persist beyond the crisis.

Building on this discussion, the following section examines six key characteristics that define how CG operates in contexts of weak state capacity, highlighting the specific ways in which these dynamics unfold across the cases analyzed. These characteristics challenge the assumptions in much of the CG literature, which presupposes stable institutions and long-term government engagement (Ansell & Gash, 2008; Emerson & Tina, 2015). Instead, our findings suggest that in Latin America, CG is shaped by political and social conditions that favor dynamic, informal, and often temporary collaborative arrangements.

7.3.1 Collaborative Governance Takes the Form of Ad Hoc Arrangements

CG in Latin America is not the same as that seen and theorized in Europe or the United States. In the region, political institutions and organizations tend to have a lower degree of institutionalization, fewer resources and inspire low levels of public trust (as further explored below). This, combined with other characteristics such as high electoral volatility, the lack of re-election, pronounced political instability, and widespread corruption (Vian, 2008), makes institutionalizing CG relationships difficult. Changes and instabilities in political positions negatively impact predictability regarding what can be done and whether there will be resources to do so. In Guatemala, for example, no single political party has achieved the presidency more than once. In Peru, political parties are so weak that power is dispersed among individuals, impeding coordination (Barrenechea & Vergara, 2023). Under these circumstances, where formal power is dispersed and de facto, extra-constitutional, powers are potentially quite influential and CG of any kind is highly disincentivized. In other words, we speak less of CG regimes and more of CG *arrangements* in Latin America.

Regimes, theorized from the evidence of the United States and Europe, are "institutionalized" governance systems where the different parties, including at least one level of government, are bound by norms and regulations created to define the initial collaborative task and guide future interactions. In other words, a collaboration regime involves stability, commitment among the parties, and regulated periodic interactions (Emerson & Tina, 2015). In contrast, arrangements are instances where different actors come together to collaborate in response to an urgent and complex problem, but these actors do not necessarily—and typically do not—dedicate efforts (time and resources) to formalize or institutionalize the collaboration over time. As a result, the collaborative arrangements identified in the region are dynamic and short-term, which, after addressing an urgent need, tend to disappear or remain latent in the face of a potential future crisis. Due to this, one of the greatest benefits of CG models—i.e., their ability to address more complex and even structural societal problems—was largely not materialized.

In Chile, for example, community collaboration among neighbors, NGOs, and other territorial organizations replaced the absent state, thanks to the redirection of experiences and the rearticulation of networks formed during the so-called "Estallido Social"[2] (2019) toward the new needs arising from the pandemic. "Ollas Comunes"[3] were a typical case of this type of collaboration. However, the great difficulty of this form of CG was its ability to sustain itself once the strictest lockdowns and restrictions were lifted.

7.3.2 *Limited National Government Participation*

In crisis contexts that require rapid responses to urgent problems, a central authority with the hierarchical capacity to coordinate resources is necessary while also leveraging the collaborative network to share information (Asuntos del Sur, 2023; Ran & Qi, 2018). This need arises from the lack of time required to establish a collaborative agreement regarding the power structure, compounded by the reluctance of the involved actors to assume the burden of responsibility. This resistance is also influenced by the associated costs, as assuming such responsibility entails exposure to potential criticism or negative consequences if the response is inadequate or insufficient.

The state's role becomes central in CG, especially in contexts of urgent needs. The cases studied for this analysis highlight the disparity of power between the actors involved or affected by a given problem, and among them, the fundamental role of the state due to its resources and territorial reach, as well as its specific obligations, competencies, and powers to guarantee access to and exercise of rights, implement public policies, and distribute public goods. Therefore, the state is a fundamental actor, and its presence or absence influences the characteristics and the likelihood of success of the collaboration. Some theoretical approaches even argue that the participation of the national government is necessarily involved when conceptualizing the phenomenon (Ansell & Gash, 2008). However, taking into account the six countries analyzed, this view is not applicable to Latin America. In fact, most of the detected CG examples did not involve the government in any way.

In all the countries examined, there is a marked tension between two issues: on one hand, the essential role that the national government can play in making a CG arrangement more effective, and on the other hand, the widespread lack of trust

---

[2] At the end of 2019 a series of protests took place in Chile in response to the structural social inequality inherited from the neoliberal model established by the *de facto* government led by Augusto Pinochet in 1973. The protests were inherently civic, as all political parties have been involved in the perpetuation of this socioeconomic model. The outbreak led to a process of constitutional reform.

[3] The Ollas Comunes emerged during the Estallido Social as a 'community kitchen' for those who had no food. They were organized by neighbors (mostly women) through donations and the purchase of food boxes.

from the citizens toward the government, particularly regarding its commitment and capacity to assist the communities that need it.

Nevertheless, despite citizens' distrust and disbelief, the government's role can be crucial for collaboration in at least three aspects:

1. Resources, including personnel, expertise, and money: These resources can be key for institutionalizing a CG arrangement.
2. The government can help extend the impact of collaboration across a territory. This occurred, for example, in Chile, where the government identified the value of a program, *Centinela Renca*, created in one municipality and used its resources to extend its reach to other municipalities.
3. The government can be a source of political will and commitment. When the government remains committed to a collaborative arrangement, it is possible for other stakeholders to "buy in" to the project as well. Indeed, in all six countries, non-governmental participants expressed authentic disbelief regarding the government's commitment to collaborate.

One of the historical challenges in Latin America has been the lack of trust from society toward political institutions. For example, data from the Latinobarómetro show declining support for various central institutions. Table 7.1 illustrates how, in all cases, the percentage of citizens distrusting these institutions was higher in 2020 than in 2000. This results in actors who share certain objectives with the government being reluctant to collaborate with it, despite these shared goals (Robertson, 2011).

The six case studies show that this significant lack of trust prevents non-state actors from wanting to participate when it comes to collaborating with the national or even local government (see Kapucu & Garayev, 2011). Why invest energy, time, and resources in forging some form of collaboration mechanism with government authorities if past experiences show they lack the power, motivation, resources, and incentives to implement a more CG approach? This aspect was highlighted by members of local communities in Bolivia, Chile, Guatemala, and Mexico.

The lack of trust in the government, compounded by its historical inability to commit to long-term collaborative mechanisms, has forced non-state local actors to create their own collaborative arrangements to compensate for these shortcomings. This occurred in all the countries covered in the study. This finding aligns with

Table 7.1 Percentage of the Latin American public with little or no trust in political institutions

	Year		
Institution	2000	2015	2020
Presidency	61%	57%	68%
Congress	72%	72%	80%
Political Parties	80%	80%	87%

Source: Latinobarómetro (2000, 2015, 2020)

recent research on Brazil and the United States (Bizzo & Michener, 2023).[4] Indeed, we found that social organizations are the main drivers of local collaboration initiatives in several countries, notably Chile, Colombia, Guatemala, and Mexico. However, community collaborative arrangements without state support were more unstable, shorter in duration, and primarily addressed urgent needs. From the perspective of Interactive Governance, the absence of the State is not a neutral feature but rather a governance deficit (Pierre & Peters, 2005). Essential state functions, such as the articulation of priorities, are missing, leaving a gap that, while local initiatives may be valuable, they cannot fill at scale.

For example, social collaboration in Mexico was necessary to influence and demand action from an absent government that failed to meet its obligations, but it was also a crucial—and necessary—actor in responding to the urgent needs of domestic workers and migrants.

However, it is important to emphasize that when the government has fully engaged in collaborative arrangements, the results for communities have been positive. For instance, in the Buenos Aires province, Argentina, the participation of the Tres de Febrero municipality allowed for the enhancement of food assistance in community kitchens at the time of greatest demand with the "Más Comunidad"[5] program. By providing a debit card instead of food products, the government was able to serve all community kitchens simultaneously, allowing them to purchase from their trusted suppliers, regulate food quantities, and take advantage of offers. In Bolivia, collaboration between the municipality of El Alto and trade organizations was key for market vendors to maintain their work, ensuring certain biosecurity measures—guaranteed by the municipality—such as permanent disinfection and vaccination as a requirement for enabling the market. This was the case with the examples of *Detectar* in Argentina, *Renca Centinela* in Chile, and the *Pacifico Task Force* in Colombia—three CG initiatives that are considered in detail in the chapters below. All three collaborative arrangements helped provide information, protective gear, and testing Covid-19 reporting capabilities to communities in need. The government was a key actor in expanding the scope and depth of each program.

At the same time, CG initiatives that include the government can produce positive feedback for participating government officials. The case studies in Chile demonstrate that, where municipal governments engaged with non-state actors in their COVID-19 policy responses, the mayor was re-elected in the following election. Collaboration can be a positive for governments that choose to work with and listen to other stakeholders.

---

[4] Bizzo and Michener (2023) consider the emergence of compensatory collaborative governance in Brazil and the United States, in response to the COVID-19 pandemic. It is notable that they link CCG with the specific, concerted efforts by presidents—specifically, Jair Bolsonaro in Brazil and Donald Trump in the United States—to deny the severity of the COVID-19 pandemic. Our point goes beyond the efforts of any single leader and instead addresses the longstanding lack of confidence in political institutions more general—which makes non-state actors less willing, in general, to work with the state when it comes to addressing community problems/demands.

[5] The Más Comunidad Program was launched in September 2020 and implemented in January 2021. There were no similar programs in other municipalities, and the idea stemmed from the Más Familias card, a municipal program implemented in 2018.

However, just as there were cases of "genuine" participation, there were also instances where government authorities made more superficial engagement, attempting to exploit the benefits of CG, mainly to achieve a positive public image, without real collaboration with non-state actors.

7.3.3 Context Matters

The potential and nature of collaboration will manifest in one way or another depending on the political and social context in which it arises and develops (Bryson et al., 2006). We identify two contextual factors that influence the form that CG takes in practice. While these are not the only factors, they are the most significant.

One of these factors is the level of trust or credibility in institutions, which, as previously explained, affects the likelihood of collaborations emerging with government authorities, along with the advantages that such collaborations imply.

The other main factor is related to historical legacies and old power relations. The postcolonial context in which Latin American states were born significantly restricted the formation of effective state institutions (Mahoney, 2010). Over time, this has hindered relations between the state and society, making it more difficult for the state to reach and care for all communities within its borders. Moreover, more recently, the region's weak states have been particularly affected by the arrival of foreign criminal organizations or gangs. These realities influence who has access to state resources and how collaborations with the state can take place (see Blofield et al., 2020). Certainly, the longstanding types of relationships also affect how different non-state actors operate and interact among themselves and with the state. In sum, we must situate present-day collaboration initiatives within the broader framework of longstanding trends that define and condition social relations.

The CG arrangements studied have been conditioned by the political and social situation. The context that preceded the arrival of Covid-19 was highly varied across the region and influenced how collaborations were formed to address the pandemic. Some countries, such as Bolivia[6] and Chile,[7] have recently undergone intense social

[6] The results of the general elections on October 20th, 2019, triggered protests, mainly from the middle classes, across the country due to suspicions of electoral fraud. More than a month after intense social conflicts, then-President Evo Morales and Vice President Álvaro García Linera resigned from their positions. On November 12th, opposition Senator Jeanine Áñez assumed the interim presidency of Bolivia, with the mandate to call for elections. However, the confrontations escalated, and a new period of conflicts began. Days after the installation of the new government, a series of mobilizations broke out in various parts of the country. The repression of the mobilized sectors was violent and carried out by the Armed Forces, who made disproportionate use of force under the protection of Supreme Decree 4078/2019, which absolved the military of any responsibility (Montes, 2021). The atmosphere of conflict between the unelected government of President Áñez and sectors of civil society remained tense throughout Áñez's year in power, which coincided with the emergence of Covid-19.

[7] See footnote 2.

and political crises that have shaped the possibilities of cross-group collaboration. While in Chile, the 2019 *Estallido Social* led to the creation of community collaboration networks that later transformed to respond to Covid-19, in Bolivia, during the de facto government led by Áñez, it was more difficult to establish dialogue between informal workers' organizations and the state, compounded by heavy street militarization. In Argentina, by contrast, the pandemic hit just as a new presidential term began. These political dynamics immediately preceding the pandemic's onset will likely shape who can participate in collaboration and how it may occur.

7.3.4 Diversity of Actors

Another key feature of the initiatives studied is the diversity of actors involved and the different modes of interaction among them. In the case of a wicked problem, for instance, ensuring the rights of migrants in transit during a pandemic, there are various actors and sectors involved, each potentially having different interests that lead to a collaborative arrangement. Regarding modes of interaction, collaborative arrangements were found involving state participation among different levels of government (multilevel, vertical, or horizontal collaboration), between a certain state level and civil society (public–private or inter-institutional collaboration), and without state involvement (social, community, or organic collaboration).

The constellation of actors who participate (or do not) in a collaboration has an impact on how that collaboration manifests and its potential success, as they bring distinct knowledge, resources, and also different interests when coming together to work collaboratively with other actors and sectors.

If most of the relevant actors involved share interests and contribute resources, then it is more likely that the solutions proposed collaboratively will be more effective, and in the long term, positive externalities could arise, even in other areas. An example is the Centinela Renca program in Chile, where local government and private national and international actors collaborated to design software for tracking Covid-19 cases. The successful results of the program encouraged collaboration with other municipalities, including some that had no prior interaction before the pandemic, leading to the adoption of the program by other governments.

On the other hand, if a collaborative arrangement lacks the participation of a key actor, such as the state or community, and thus lacks their resources and expertise, the collaboration will be partial, its results, while positive, will be limited, and it will face greater obstacles in terms of formalization and long-term sustainability.

In Argentina, for instance, during the health emergency, a community-based collaborative initiative emerged among public schools that offered their facilities and volunteers to manage the distribution of donated food. However, it was a very short-lived experience that quickly dissipated, as without state support or resources, the CG arrangement became unsustainable: donations ran out, and volunteers ceased participating due to contracting the disease.

Finally, if mutual distrust prevails in a collaboration initiative and there is no willingness to share resources or work together toward a common goal, dynamics of competition are likely to arise, or each actor may implement parallel actions, leading to confusion and neutralizing positive impacts, or the collaboration may end without achieving any effective solution. This type of collaborative dynamic occurred in Mexico when, due to the change in leadership at the National Human Rights Commission (CNDH), the interests of this actor shifted, and because they differed from those of the Migratory Policy Working Group (a civil society and university network for the rights of migrant populations in transit), previous agreements could not be implemented. A similar situation occurred in the Argentine municipality of Tres de Febrero, where the mayor and the provincial governor belonged to different parties and were in opposition at both the provincial and national levels. This confrontation limited the possibilities for multilevel collaboration in implementing the vaccination campaign, resulting in a disorganized and fragmented campaign. Although competition did not escalate, it increased future coordination costs and widened the structural differences between municipalities, even adjacent ones.

7.3.5 Short-Term and Dynamic

In Latin America, CG arrangements are predominantly short-term and dynamic. While some institutionalized examples existed before the Covid-19 outbreak and were adapted to address the pandemic, most lacked formal structures. Institutionalized collaborations tended to have clearer regulations and participation rules, but these were the exception rather than the norm.

In general, the cases analyzed revealed that CG emerged as ad hoc arrangements, formed in response to specific needs within particular contexts. A key factor behind this lack of institutionalization was the limited participation of the government, as discussed earlier. Without sustained state involvement, these collaborations had fewer resources to develop long-term mechanisms. Additionally, the widespread lack of trust in collaborative processes, combined with the financial and operational constraints of community organizations and other non-state actors, further hindered their ability to transition into enduring governance structures.

As a result, the CG arrangements observed in the region shared two defining characteristics: they were highly dynamic and short-lived.

First, they exhibited a fluid and evolving nature. Actors who initially spearheaded a collaboration often withdrew over time, while new participants joined at different stages. Government officials, in particular, were prone to inconsistent engagement, with their involvement fluctuating due to political changes or shifting priorities (Blair & Janousek, 2013). For example, in Argentina and Chile, we found cases of collaborations that began with the participation of government agents who later withdrew. In these cases, the collaborations had a markedly vertical nature from the start: the state joined local agents to address a specific need. These structures became more horizontal after the government withdrew its support. At that point, new non-state actors were incorporated to replace the government. In other cases, it was found that the government joined already existing collaboration initiatives. An example was the *Centinela Renca* program in Chile. The initiative was successful, and over time, the government joined to develop the program further and expand it to other municipalities.

One of these dynamic cases was the *Preicfes Comunitario Paulo Freire* initiative, which provided pedagogical tools to prepare for the test granting access to Colombia's higher education. Thanks to the collaboration between grassroots organizations, families, leaders, university professors, and the community in general, who articulated various strategies such as food distribution, internet plans, and psychosocial support, school dropout rates were reduced, and test scores improved. Due to this success, government entities from the country and international organizations like the Colombian Institute for the Evaluation of Education and the German Embassy joined the initiative.

Another example of this relationship is the Pacific Task Force alliance, which brought together academia, civil society organizations, and local governments to develop strategic actions that helped mitigate the vulnerability exacerbated by Covid-19 in the Pacific region of Colombia. Although civil society organizations and academia initiated it, other relevant actors, such as municipal governments, local government secretariats, and educational institutions, joined during the implementation process. Thus, from an ethnic-racial and intersectional perspective, the multilevel collaboration arrangement allowed information to be provided and to map needs and opportunities for complementarity between the public, private, and community sectors.

The dynamic nature of collaboration in Latin America allows for a certain amount of flexibility when dealing with pressing needs, to be sure (Kapucu & Garayev, 2011). Nevertheless, where the collaborative arrangement can potentially change from one day to the next, it is more difficult to set expectations regarding how collaboration occurs. Stakeholders may doubt others' commitment to the collaborative arrangement. Levels of influence may vary. Other factors—including political pressures, asymmetrical access to resources, and/or self-interest—may erode confidence in collaboration's potential. In short, the dynamic nature of collaboration in Latin America may actually weaken the incentives to collaborate and, consequently, hamper the possibility of institutionalization in the future.[8]

A second feature of the CG arrangements analyzed was that they tended to be short-term in extension. As pandemic-related problems emerged, actors came together to address that problem collaboratively. The collaborative effort would dissipate once the problem was addressed sufficiently, or to the extent possible. In practice, this meant that most of the collaborative responses that we examine below focused on a need for, for instance, food, masks, medicine, tests, or information.

Certainly, addressing the immediate needs generated by the pandemic was not an easy task, as communities and their territories had already been facing structural issues of scarcity before the Covid-19 outbreak. The pandemic exacerbated these deficiencies. Additionally, it introduced one or more new causes of illness and death. Lockdown policies increased the precariousness of these communities' economies.

---

[8] For more on the importance of institutionalization in managing urgent crises, see Lu (2017).

The pandemic brought to light the serious material problems that groups in situations of vulnerability face. These problems, of course, are symptomatic of much more deeply rooted issues: poverty, inequality, inequity, racism, and sexism. The collaborative arrangements in Latin America tended to be dynamic and short-lived. As a result, one of the key advantages of CG—its potential to tackle complex and deeply rooted societal challenges—remained largely unrealized.

7.3.6 Power Asymmetries and (Lack of) Representativeness

Short-term collaborative arrangements can be sensitive to the disproportionate influence of actors with more resources, time, or energy to engage in collaboration. A recurring concern was the asymmetries between and within the working groups. For example, it is expected that the private sector will have more resources at its disposal than civil society organizations. Additionally, some civil society organizations have better contacts or more access routes than other parties.

This raises a question about the undemocratic or unrepresentative nature of collaboration initiatives. While these asymmetries in the capacity to influence are not new regarding CG (Carboni et al., 2017), their impact can be more pronounced in countries where asymmetries between parties are intertwined with state bureaucracies and political institutions that are highly politicized. Therefore, CG models in a region like Latin America may not only fail to address the structural inequalities between groups and within them, but they may also reproduce and exacerbate them. In line with the Faustian bargain (Pierre & Peters, 2005), a weak State—lacking either the capacity or the will to engage a broad range of actors—may choose to negotiate only with the most organized or powerful groups, while ignoring those who are more vulnerable or underrepresented.

For example, in Bolivia, the state called on union leaders without considering that representatives are often men, even though 85.7% of self-employed workers are women (OIT, ONU Mujeres, & PNUD, 2022). This lack of representativeness and inclusion of female union leaders had tangible effects on their lives, as no specific actions were designed to address the risks they faced during the strict quarantine.

7.4 Conclusions

Collaborative governance (CG) in Latin America during the Covid-19 pandemic proved to be a highly relevant tool for addressing complex problems. The collaborative arrangements differ from those observed in the Global North. In Latin America, where institutions are often weak, resources scarce, and trust in government limited, CG took on specific forms: dynamic, short-term arrangements that emerged as ad hoc responses to urgent needs rather than as formalized regimes.

However, when collaboration occurred, the results were very positive. The cases analyzed in Argentina, Bolivia, Chile, Colombia, Guatemala, and Mexico demonstrate that collaboration between state and non-state actors allowed for addressing the immediate demands of the health, economic, and social crises. However, the lack of institutionalization and structural distrust among the actors limited the scope of these collaborations, hindering their long-term sustainability and ability to address structural inequalities.

Specifically, the analysis highlighted the importance of the state as a key actor in enhancing collaborative arrangements. Its participation can provide resources, legitimacy, and territorial reach. Yet, the absence of the government was a constant in many of the documented experiences, leaving civil society organizations and other local actors responsible for compensating for these gaps, often resulting in limited and fragmented responses. The role assumed by the government has serious implications for the potential of CG and will be an important point to explore in future research concerning the CG agenda and its functioning in the Global South. While collaboration has been an indispensable tool for survival, its manifestation in Latin America reveals a deep deficit in state capacity and democratic legitimacy. The challenge moving forward is not only to promote collaboration, but to rebuild the role of the State as a guarantor of inclusive and accountable governance.

Looking ahead, it is essential to deepen the understanding of how these dynamics could be institutionalized to turn CG arrangements into institutionalized, sustainable, and long-term regimes capable of addressing not only emerging crises but also the structural problems that characterize the region. Ultimately, the pandemic highlighted the transformative potential of CG but also its limits. Leveraging these lessons can undoubtedly allow CG to be used as a strategic tool to improve public policy quality, legitimacy, and sustainability. Future research on CG in Latin America should consider a broader range of theoretical models, including Interactive Governance (Torfing et al., 2012) framework, to better capture the diversity and fragility of collaborative arrangements in low-capacity states.

References

Ansell, C., & Gash, A. (2008). Collaborative governance in theory and practice. *Journal of Public Administration Research and Theory, 18*(4), 543–571. Oxford Academic.

Asuntos del Sur. (2023). *Cómo Gobernar Colaborativamente.* https://asuntosdelsur.org/wp-content/uploads/2023/11/PolicyRecomendations_ColaboraLat.pdf

Barandiarán, X., Canel, M. J., & Bouckaert, G. (2022). ¿Qué mueve a confiar en la gobernanza colaborativa? Análisis de un programa gubernamental en el País Vasco. *Revista Española de Ciencia Política, 60*, 251–275. https://doi.org/10.21308/recp.60.09

Barrenechea, R., & Vergara, A. (2023). El vaciamiento democrático en Perú… y más allá. *Nueva Sociedad.*

Bennett, S., Glandon, D., & Rasanathan, K. (2018). Governing multisectoral action for health in low-income and middle-income countries: Unpacking the problem and rising to the challenge. *BMJ Global Health, 3*(Suppl 4), e000880.

Bianchi, C., Nasi, G., & Rivenbark, W. C. (2021). Implementing collaborative governance: Models, experiences, and challenges. *Public Management Review, 23*(11), 1581–1589. https://doi.org/10.1080/14719037.2021.1878777
Bizzo, E., & Michener, G. (2023). Compensatory collaborative governance: Filling pandemic transparency gaps in Brazil and the United States. *Public Management Review*, 1–26.
Blair, R., & Janousek, C. L. (2013). Collaborative mechanisms in interlocal cooperation: A longitudinal examination. *State and Local Government Review, 45*(4), 268–282.
Blofield, M., Hoffmann, B., & Llanos, M. (2020). Assessing the Political and Social Impact of the COVID-19 Crisis in Latin America. (GIGA Focus Lateinamerika, 3). Hamburg: GIGA German Institute of Global and Area Studies – Leibniz-Institut für Globale und Regionale Studien, Institut für Lateinamerika-Studien. https://nbn-resolving.org/urn:nbn:de:0168-ssoar-67260-7
Bryson, J. M., Crosby, B. C., & Stone, M. M. (2006). The design and implementation of cross-sector collaborations: Propositions from the literature. *Public Administration Review, 66*(1), 44–55.
Carboni, J. L., Siddiki, S., Koski, C., & Sadiq, A. A. (2017). Using network analysis to identify key actors in collaborative governance processes. In A. Abramson, S. Toepler, & M. Kim (Eds.), *Nonprofit policy forum* (pp. 133–145). De Gruyter.
Colabora.Lat. (2022). *Índice de Gobernanza Colaborativa.* Recuperado de https://colabora.lat/indice/#:~:text=El%20%C3%8Dndice%20de%20Gobernanza%20Colaborativa,pol%C3%ADticas%20frente%20al%20covid%2D19
Comisión Económica para América Latina y el Caribe (CEPAL). (2021). *Informe sobre el impacto del COVID-19 en América Latina y el Caribe.*
Cyr, J., Bianchi, M., González, L., & Perini, A. (2021). Governing a Pandemic: Assessing the role of collaboration on Latin American responses to the COVID-19 crisis. *Journal of Politics in Latin America, 13*(3), 290–327. https://doi.org/10.1177/1866802X211049250
Cyr, J., Bianchi, M., Coda, F., & Santamarina, S. (Eds.) (2025). *Repensando la gobernanza en América Latina. La colaboración como herramienta para afrontar los desafíos del siglo XXI.* Fondo de Cultura Económica.
Emerson, K., & Nabatchi, T. (2015). *Collaborative governance regimes.* Georgetown University Press.
Kapucu, N., & Garayev, V. (2011). Collaborative decision-making in emergency and disaster management. *International Journal of Public Administration, 34*(6), 366–375.
Latinobarómetro (2000, 2015 y 2020). Informes disponibles en https://www.latinobarometro.org/latContents.jsp.
Lu, X. (2017). *Managing uncertainty in crisis: Exploring the impact of institutionalization on organizational sensemaking* (1st ed.). Springer Nature.
Mahoney, J. (2010). *Colonialism and postcolonial development: Spanish America in comparative perspective.* Cambridge University Press.
Montes, T. (2021). Feminismos de la ciudad de El Alto: Una visión desde los colectivos. El Alto: Centro de Promoción de la Mujer "Gregoria Apaza", OXFAM.
OIT, ONU Mujeres, & PNUD. (2022). Caracterización de mujeres cuentapropistas informales en Bolivia: Estudio comprensivo. (1st ed.). La Paz: Organización Internacional del Trabajo, Oficina de la OIT para los Países Andinos, [ONU Mujeres, Programa de Naciones Unidas para el Desarrollo].
Pierre, J., & Peters, B. G. (2005). *Governing complex societies: Trajectories and scenarios.* Palgrave Macmillan.
Ran, B., & Qi, H. (2018). Gobernanza colaborativa: Las contingencias del poder compartido. *Estado abierto, 2*(3), 47–90.
Rittel, H. W. J., & Webber, M. M. (1973). Dilemmas in a general theory of planning. *Policy Sciences, 4*(2), 155–169.
Robertson, P. J. (2011). An assessment of collaborative governance in a network for sustainable tourism: The case of RedeTuris. *International Journal of Public Administration, 34*(5), 279–290.

Rodríguez, L., & Ortiz, M. (2021). *La importancia del servicio civil en el desarrollo de capacidades estatales en América Latina*. Academia.edu.
Torfing, J., Peters, B. G., Pierre, J., & Sørensen, E. (2012). *Interactive governance: Advancing the paradigm*. Oxford University Press.
Ulibarri, N., Imperial, M. T., Siddiki, S., & Henderson, H. (2023). Drivers and dynamics of collaborative governance in environmental management. *Environmental Management, 71*, 495–504. https://doi.org/10.1007/s00267-022-01769-7
UNESCO. (2020). *Global Education Monitoring Report 2020 – Latin America and the Caribbean – Inclusion and education: All means all*. UNESCO.
Vian, T. (2008). Review of corruption in the health sector: Theory, methods and interventions. *Health Policy and Planning, 23*(2), 83–94. https://doi.org/10.1093/heapol/czm048
World Bank. (2024). *Innovating bureaucracy for a more capable government*. Banco Mundial.

Chapter 8
State Capacities in Argentina's COVID-19 Vaccine Endeavor: Challenges, Strategies, and Lessons Toward Pandemic Preparedness

María Cecilia Sanmartín and Gabriela Bortz

> "Never in [the country's] history has there been such a massive and widespread vaccination, which is a logistical, operational, and scheduling challenge of an unprecedented magnitude." (Ministry of Health, 2023)

> "If we had not had a flag carrier, I don't know if we would have managed to bring in what we brought those first months of the pandemic." (Ministry of Health, 2023).

8.1 Introduction

How did the Argentine state—amid a new ruling coalition, a fragmented health system, deep socio-political divides, empty federal reserves, and a peripheral position in global value chains— manage to align and coordinate capacities to confront the COVID-19 pandemic? This chapter addresses this question by analyzing how the Argentine state acquired, produced, developed, and delivered COVID-19 vaccines to its citizenship. Healthcare technologies—ranging from diagnostic reagents and masks to, most notably, vaccines—reasserted their political significance as symbols of state policy (Joerges, 1999) and as political technologies shaping national imaginaries and the state's envisioned role (Winner, 1993).

Although the first COVID-19 case in Argentina was reported in Buenos Aires on March 3, 2020 (Ministry of Health, 2020), the government declared the national health emergency on March 19 (Boletín Oficial, 2020). This positioned the state as a central actor while testing its historical capacity to protect public health (Arce, 2010). In this pressing context, vaccines emerged as a great promise for addressing the global health crisis. Major pharmaceutical companies worldwide raised expectations about vaccine development, intensifying efforts for market capture

M. C. Sanmartín (✉) · G. Bortz
Universidad Nacional de San Martin, National Council of Scientific and Technical Research (CONICET), San Martin, Argentina

I. Okada (ed.), *COVID-19 and State Capacity in Latin America*, Latin American Societies, https://doi.org/10.1007/978-3-032-15572-6_8

(Balajewder et al., 2021; Zhang, 2021). However, vaccine research and development (R&D) and manufacturing remained concentrated in developed countries—the global "center"—widening geopolitical and access disparities with the "periphery" (Blinder et al., 2021; Sanmartin, 2023).

In Argentina, health is a constitutional right (Art. 42), and healthcare products are treated as social goods (Santos & Thomas, 2018). The country also has the most comprehensive National Vaccination Calendar in the region and one of the world's highest rates of vaccine confidence (94% in 2019) (Fundación Bunge & Born, 2021). It also presents a long national trajectory of biomedical and clinical research and over four decades of excellence in health biotechnology R&D (Kreimer & Thomas, 2005; Kreimer, 2010; Romero, 2016). These capabilities helped consolidate a dynamic ecosystem of biotechnology companies (Stubrin, 2022).

However, the planning and implementation of Argentina's COVID-19 Immunization Program in late 2020 and 2021 were shaped by both existing state capacities and a challenging geopolitical and economic context. Amid chronic crises—42% inflation, 40.6% poverty, and rising social unrest—a newly elected, heterogeneous coalition faced internal tensions and fragmented leadership at different state levels (Andrenacci, 2023; Caravaca & Daniel, 2023). Coordination was further complicated by Argentina's mixed and decentralized healthcare system, where provinces and municipalities hold autonomy over health policy and logistics, challenging a coordinated national pandemic response (Maceira, 2020; Marin, 2021; Gollan et al., 2021). This decentralization also extended to the logistics of mandatory vaccination campaigns (Olin, 2018). Additionally, although Argentina has strong Science, Technology, and Innovation (STI) capacities, they often remained disconnected from local needs, leading to dependence on imported biotechnological vaccines.

During the pandemic, Argentina implemented emergency economic and welfare policies for vulnerable households and the private sector, alongside confinement and circulation restrictions[1] (Heredia, 2022; Caravaca & Daniel, 2023). Specifically, vaccine procurement, distribution, production, and development triggered an unprecedented realignment among government agencies, federal councils, research units, public labs, and local industries. Drawing on strong biomedical, biotechnological, and clinical research techno-scientific capacities, Argentina became a testing hub for COVID-19 vaccines developed by major global biopharmaceutical companies. While scientific, industrial, and regulatory capabilities enabled securing agreements for vaccine component manufacturing, aiding the pandemic response in 2021, these also allowed Argentina to become in 2023 the first Latin American country to fully develop a COVID-19 vaccine approved by an internationally recognized regulator (Sanmartin & Bortz, 2024). These actions relied on flexible articulation across institutions and capacities, led by the Ministry of Health and the public

[1] For instance, certain containment measures in the Metropolitan Buenos Aires Area intensified reinforced existing policies that segregated and isolated slums during crises.

STI sector, to engage scientific and private actors in coalitions based on cognitive, symbolic, and material elements.

This chapter analyzes how Argentine state agencies mobilized resources, technologies, knowledge, and coordination mechanisms to secure vaccine access during the pandemic. It explores how the state tackled the logistical, operational, and implementation challenges of an unprecedented vaccination campaign, and how the state of exception activated latent state capacities that redefined the state's role during a crisis. We argue for including the symbolic dimension into state capacity analysis, understanding how historical imaginaries shape actors' decisions and expectations rooted in pre-existing institutional resources, capacities, and beliefs.

This study draws on a qualitative methodology, including 37 interviews with key actors in COVID-19 national dynamics (government, scientists, science advisors, and private sector representatives) and documentary analysis of 150 newspaper articles published between March 2020 and August 2023, exploring the media's role in shaping public perceptions. The analysis focuses on the discursive repertoires of actors from the national government, health and scientific sectors, and the local biopharmaceutical industry. Using an inductive, constructivist grounded theory approach, we iteratively connected empirical data and theory to identify key themes in the interplay of meaning, power, and inequality (Charmaz, 2016).

Argentina's quest to gain access to COVID-19 vaccines highlighted the critical role of the state, its capacities, and key actors in strategic coordination positions. We argue that state capabilities, although constrained by national circumstances, were driven by symbolic representations of the state's role, rooted in the government coalition's vision of what was possible and desirable. Amid tensions between sovereignty aspirations and perceptions of peripheral dependence, the sovereignty narrative helped realign actors and mobilize capacities across a fragmented state apparatus to (re)construct its role in securing vaccine access. This chapter is structured as follows: Section 8.2 reviews literature on state capacities, including perspectives from the social studies of technology. Section 8.3 provides a historical view connecting state capacities with collective representations of the state's role in health and STI. Section 8.4 analyzes how vaccine acquisition, production, and development redefined capacities, framing access through a sovereignty-dependence narrative that casts the state as a welfare guarantor enacted through vaccines and vaccination.

8.2 State Capacities: Political Agency, Knowledge, and Imaginaries

The concept of state capacity, rooted in debates on the state's role in development, has evolved alongside changing conceptions of state's function (Ottervik, 2013). Various frameworks capture its policy implementation ability, including state power

(Skocpol, 1979; Mann, 1984; Tilly, 1991), state strength (Migdal, 2004), state capacity (Fukuyama, 2013), and government effectiveness (Rothstein, 2011).

This chapter follows the state capacity definition as elaborated in Chap. 1, assuming it as the capacity of the state to implement political decisions. This aligns with what Migdal (1988) defines: state capacity as the ability of state leaders to use state agencies to shape societal behavior and drive change through policies and planning: "get people in society to do what they want them to do" or "to bring about the types of changes in society that their leaders seek through planning, policies, and state actions." In this chapter, we specifically consider how the state utilizes power and political apparatus to orchestrate diverse ideologies and interests across sectors while managing material and human resources within the public sphere. As Besley (2006) suggests, political agency requires balancing particular interests with collective goals to avoid clientelism or private capture. For Hameiri (2007), state capacities emerge from conflicts, power struggles, institutional trajectories, and the interests they advance or resist.

Drawing from innovation economics, long-term capabilities emerge through cumulative learning and path-dependence, locking decisions into specific trajectories and creating irreversibility (David, 1994; Callon, 1990). Distinguishing state capacity from political decisions, the former aligns resources and institutions, laying the groundwork for future action under evolving conditions—what Blofield et al. (2023) call "policy legacies." These are shaped by existing knowledge, organizational structures, and cultural norms. While structural constraints matter, agency that transforms political decisions into implementation plays a key role in shaping concrete policy design and implementation, often exposing institutional fragilities and susceptibility to political influence (Corrales, 2018; Geddes, 1994). Thus, state capacity focuses on the action and interaction between state and social actors operating in specific institutional and structural environments (Amengual & Dargent, 2020). In this sense, Weiss and Thurbon (2022) suggest that state agents' decisions can mitigate institutional weaknesses that might otherwise have been critical, activate latent capacities, or, conversely, or undermine strategies entirely prompting a change in direction.

While political science has often overlooked Science, Technology, and Innovation (STI) policies (Jasanoff, 2004), these not only constitute a specific area of governance but also serve broader political, socio-economic, and strategic goals. Recent work highlights the state's role in steering technological change to tackle complex challenges (Mazzucato, 2011, 2018; Schot & Steinmueller, 2018). This shift challenges pro-market and managerial views that reduced the state's role to addressing market failures, leading to outsourcing and capability loss (Ezrahi, 1990) and confining the state to a facilitator role. These studies argue that losing capabilities makes the state slow and ineffective, creating the same self-fulfilling prophecy of inefficiency it seeks to escape.

These approaches emphasize the central role of bureaucracies in building state capabilities. In a Neo-Weberian revisitation, Kattel et al. (2022) argue that effective policy and innovation governance depends on "agile stability"—a balance between flexible dynamic networks and stable expert institutions. This allows bureaucracies to remain dynamic and change-responsive, capable of translating innovation policies into actionable programs, managing resources, coordinating stakeholders, and resilient in achieving long-term goals across political changes. They provide the required institutional expertise for sustained policies, ensuring continuity, adaptive learning, and informed decision-making in evolving contexts.

But what drives movement within these fragmented bureaucracies? This chapter argues that state capacity analysis requires frameworks that explain how policy direction and preferences and shared purpose are formed, aligning scattered state areas toward a common goal. To address this, Science, Technology, and Society (STS) studies show that ideologies and visions of the future—such as public good, justice, democracy, and sovereignty—shape policy choices and capacity trajectories (Adler, 1987; Jasanoff & Kim, 2019). Policy responses are guided not only by technical and economic demands, but also future aspirations through technology and innovation, influencing policy agenda setting, prioritizing technologies and social organizations over competing alternatives (Joly, 2010).

Sociotechnical imaginaries, rooted in local norms and values, project desirable futures and steer innovation pathways (Jasanoff & Kim, 2019). Though often originating in private visions, they gain traction through political negotiation and coalition-building (Rudek, 2022). Key political leaders play a critical role, providing not only "know-how" and "know-what" (Lundvall & Johnson, 1994) but also defining "know-where-to," setting expectations, helping define goals and policy directions. These visions of the state legitimize or challenge existing socio-political orders, shaping what state institutions can achieve with available (or achievable) resources, connections, and expertise.

8.3 The Argentine Scenario: Politics, Capacities, and Changing State Visions

Since the mid-twentieth century, the Argentine state has been positioned in a central role as a key guarantor of social rights. This includes healthcare access (Belló & Becerril-Montekio, 2011), enshrined as a constitutional right (Art. 49), and supported through free public health services (Azpiazu, 1999; Nochteff, 2001; Abrutzky et al., 2019). The country's mixed and decentralized healthcare system combines public and private supply segmented by population targets (Marin, 2021; Gollan et al., 2021). It features an extensive infrastructure network, high-complexity services, advanced technical capacity, requiring significant public spending (Spinelli, 2010). Vaccination is compulsory (Law 22.909, 1983), with the national government providing 18 free vaccines through one of the world's most comprehensive immunization calendars and achieving a 90% vaccine acceptance rate (Fundación Bunge & Born, 2021). Argentina also boasts a robust biotechnology R&D and industrial trajectory (Gutman & Lavarello, 2016; Stubrin, 2022) and a legacy of biomedical research excellence in the public sector (Kreimer, 2010; Romero, 2016).

Protectionist policies in the 1980s and limited adherence to international intellectual property regulations fostered growth in national laboratories, particularly in biosimilars and vaccines (Gutman, 2018; Amoretti, 2023). Today, domestic companies supply 70.8% of the local market and are expanding exports (CILFA, 2021). This is supported by Argentina's regulatory agency, ANMAT, recognized by the WHO as a Regional Reference Authority (MoH, 2024). Since 2010, the state has prioritized strengthening domestic manufacturing capacities of biological products to reduce public healthcare costs, address trade deficits, and promote exports (Correa et al., 2023). However, recurring cycles of growth and stagnation since the 1990s challenged sustained industry development (Naspleda, 2023).

Throughout the twentieth century, state–society relationships have been shaped by shifting political contexts and public–private dynamics (Lerner, 1988). Different authors (Adler, 1987; Lerner, 1988; Perissinotto, 2021) identify two competing national visions that intensified after the 1940s. One, a nationalist developmental project mobilized by intellectuals, envisioned an "active" and "protective state" aligned with anti-dependency ideas. This vision regarded the state as a planner and resource allocator, an economic agent driving demand to overcome dependency and foster national development (Fajnzylber, 1998; Merino, 2004; Rovere, 2004). The other, backed by landowners, conservative industrialists, and laissez-faire advocates, favored outward-oriented development, using public resources to sustain the elite while limiting popular participation (Lerner, 1988; Giraudo & Grugel, 2022). These divergent visions shaped contrasting state's roles, ranging from "developmental" to "repressive" (Lerner, 1988).

In the 1990s, there was a shift in the focus and depth of state intervention: from a state-centered to a market-centered model, with decisive but selective state intervention favoring specific actors amid sweeping market reforms (Vilas, 1997; Azpiazu, 1999; Arceo & Basualdo, 2006). Economic restructuring and state downsizing, aligned with global trends, were justified by narratives portraying the state and its bureaucracy as a "clumsy giant" unable to keep pace to rapid social, economic, and technological change (Dezalay & Garth, 2002). State reforms led to the decentralization of health and education to the subnational level, weakening national governance and raising concerns about corruption (Estévez, 2001).

After the 2001 crisis, opposing narratives challenged the "neoliberal specter" associated with an "absent state." These reframed the state's role as guarantor of public interest, democracy, and social rights, associated with discourses of national sovereignty as self-determination, opposed to foreign power dependency (La Serna, 2013). This period was marked by alternating government models: from a "modern state" focused on "austerity, efficiency, and the effective allocation of public resources" (Rosso, 2023), to one favoring greater state intervention. This oscillation, fueled by perceptions of the state becoming political booty in a divided political scene, eroded the public sector's legitimacy, undermining its ability to set norms, build consensus, and sustain institutional structures, executive functions and coordination (Madoery, 2005). This institutional fragility has been central to Argentina's political and economic instability (Levitsky & Murillo, 2005; Tommasi & Spiller, 2007).

8.4 COVID-19 Vaccines in Argentina

The COVID-19 pandemic hit Argentina amid political polarization, contested models of state-hood, and debates over the legitimacy of state intervention. The newly elected ruling coalition faced the challenge of executing health and economic policies with limited resources, particularly for vaccine procurement. After the first global vaccine candidates were announced in July 2020, the Ministry of Health began planning an immunization strategy, while navigating global competition and vaccine nationalism—high-income countries securing priority access through supply restrictions and vaccine hoarding—which deepened access inequalities for low- and middle-income countries (Vanderslott et al., 2021). As shown below, Argentina's efforts unfolded in three overlapping phases (March 2020–July 2024): acquiring imported vaccines, producing foreign-developed vaccines locally, and developing a national COVID-19 vaccine.

8.4.1 Vaccine Acquisition

In mid-2020, Argentina's Ministry of Health (MoH) initiated negotiations with multiple vaccine developers. Efforts to secure the Pfizer-BioNTech *Comirnaty* vaccine stalled over procurement terms, including upfront payments and jurisdiction waivers, sparking public concern and media scrutiny (Thomas et al., 2021; Blanco, 2020; Infobae, 2020a, 2020b; Demonte et al., 2024). During these negotiations, the government introduced the COVID-19 Vaccine Act in September 2020—passed in November—to create a legal framework for expedited procurement, bypassing regular administration procedures, enable advance payments, and strengthen the Ministry's authority during the emergency (*MoH official, personal communication, August 8,* 2023).

Amid uncertainty over vaccine availability, the MoH, the National Immunization Commission (CONAIN), and the 24 provincial health ministers debated Argentina's immunization strategy. Rising contagion risk and uncertainty enabled national authorities to lead through political negotiation and multilevel coordination, across a fragmented federal healthcare system, polarized politics, and economic crisis (Andrenacci, 2023; Neaera Abers et al., 2021).

In November 2020, amid ongoing, the government opened communications with the Russian Direct Investment Fund (RDIF) for 25 million Sputnik V doses. Key officials emphasized the importance of political leadership and personal ties in facilitating the agreement: "a very personal relationship. (...) We carried it out as individuals" (*Executive Power official, personal communication, March 15, 2024*). Argentina's strategic ties with Russia and trust built by previous governments helped prioritized negotiations (Diputados Argentina, 2021). The first 3000 doses of Sputnik V arrived on December 24, 2020 via Aerolíneas Argentinas, the flagship carrier, as many others to come, launching the vaccination campaign. The government arranged special flights and expedited customs to speed up distribution (Bortz & Sanmartin, 2023).

Argentina's COVID-19 vaccination strategy aimed to pursue bioethical principles of equality, equity, social benefit, and reciprocity based on vaccine availability (Ministry of Health, 2020; Bortz & Sanmartin, 2023). Despite existing vaccination capacities, the scale of the campaign—130% larger than previous efforts—posed major challenges amid global shortages (Comisión Técnica Asesora de Salud, 2020). The mission required enhanced operational capabilities, including: (a) securing $53 million USD for supplies, equipment acquisition—freezers and ultra-freezers—logistics and staff to manipulate diverse vaccine alternatives across the country; (b) training 36,000 vaccinators and support teams for registration, guidance, logistics, stock control, and follow-up; (c) expanding digital systems to track vaccination nationwide; (d) adapting 7749 facilities—schools, retirement centers, sports clubs, and religious establishments—to serve vaccination sites, adjusting them to health protocols; (e) and coordinating nationwide logistics, including security forces, to deliver vaccines to metropolitan areas within 12 hours and to provincial capitals within 24 (Bortz & Sanmartin, 2023).

At the ministerial level, technical teams were strengthened to turn political decisions into actions (*MoH official, personal communication, August 8,* 2023). A key initiative was the launch of the Federal Vaccination Registry (Nomivac) on March 24, 2021—an open-data platform to promote transparency and public access to vaccination progress, created to restore trust after the "VIP vaccination" scandal, where politically connected individuals bypassed the Immunization Plan's priorities. (Demonte et al., 2024). The MoH also restructured its bureaucracy to better engage local STI capabilities, creating the Comprehensive Health Risk Management Unit to coordinate emergency response (*MoH official, personal communication, August 8,* 2023).

The MoH expanded its role beyond health procurement, strengthening interministerial coordination and engaging with the productive sector. Close collaboration with ANMAT was key to fast-track vaccine emergency access under the COVID-19 Vaccine Law. ANMAT assessed documentation, issued technical reports, and adapted its rigid procedures by building technical capacity and training staff. Expert teams reviewed vaccines while training additional staff, enabling ANMAT—a traditionally procedural agency—to gain new insights, enhancing its evaluation practices, particularly for innovative products without prior approval from global reference agencies.

Local trial evaluation capacity was strengthened as ANMAT authorized phase 2/3 trials for Pfizer-BioNTech (July 2020), Sinopharm (August), and Janssen (September). Amid vaccine delays and the Delta variant surge in 2021, the MoH, the CONAIN, and expert committees assessed the immunogenicity and safety of heterologous vaccination schemes to accelerate immunization (Pasquale et al., 2022; United Nations, 2021). This aligned key actors and reinforced large-scale local trial capabilities. Though controversial, the strategy was framed by a "protective state" narrative, presenting vaccines as symbols of equitable healthcare access and sovereignty under state leadership, facing external dependence:

> I believe that this year, we have learned to value the value of a state that invests in health and science and that takes care of all Argentines. Not only is the state's intervention valued, but also the state working strongly with the private sector, strengthening Argentina's resources. (Deputy of the Justicialist Party, 9th Ordinary Session of the Chamber of Deputies, 07–10–2020)

> The state takes charge of promoting (the course) the integration of industry, the substitution of imports, and the start of post-pandemic recovery. For this purpose, the state is the flagship that will guide these different scales of companies in these national priorities. (Deputy of the Justicialist Party, 9th Ordinary Session of the Chamber of Deputies, 07–10–2020)

> Now, with the crisis, it is exacerbated in an incalculable dimension, therefore we must value this [...] if you do not have more state, your right [to health] is not guaranteed. (Former Minister of Health of PBA, Soberanía Sanitaria, 2020.)

Amid deep political divisions and distrust among the government, opposition, and media supporters (Bracco & Porta Fernández, 2022), and after months of strict lockdown, the COVID-19 immunization strategy was central to socio-economic recovery especially in urban and periurban areas, and to maintaining political stability and the ruling coalition's legitimacy.

8.4.2 *Domestic Manufacturing*

To secure COVID-19 vaccine access, Argentina pursued local production through technological transfer agreements with foreign firms. In August 2020, the Argentine-Spanish holding Insud partnered with AstraZeneca and the Slim Foundation. Under the agreement, its Argentinean-based company mAbxience—a biosimilar drug manufacturer under international standards—would produce 150–250 million doses of the Oxford/AstraZeneca vaccine's active ingredient, which would be sent to Mexico's Liomont company for formulation and packaging (Infobae, 2020b, August 12). However, supply shortages delayed the arrival of the first (partially) locally produced doses—secured through COVAX and direct talks with AstraZeneca—until May 29, 2021, during the Delta surge (Smink, 2021). In the following months, mAbxience supplied 75% of AstraZeneca's committed doses covering 24.4% of Argentina's total vaccine demand (Bortz & Sanmartin, 2023).

In January 2021, the national pharmaceutical Richmond Laboratories contacted the Russian Direct Investment Fund (RDIF) through the Indian company Hetero Labs Limited—a supplier for both parties—to produce Sputnik V locally (Infobae, 2021, February 26). Under the agreement, Richmond formulated the vaccine using active ingredients imported from Russia. Though presented as a private deal, the company acknowledged government support—especially with import logistics (La Nación, 2021). Richmond also transferred its batch analysis know-how to ANMAT, following Russian protocol guidelines.

These efforts drew on the biopharmaceutical sector's manufacturing capabilities (Lavarello et al., 2023; Stubrin, 2022), supported by a state-led scientific and technological push. Public expertise, skilled labor, and public–private funding helped build local vaccine manufacturing capabilities, driven by self-sufficiency expectations, also enabled by the capabilities developed under state intervention.

> The pandemic highlighted the region's need for self-sufficiency. (Former Health Minister, 08–02–2023)
>
> With 200 production plants, 160 nationally owned and 40 public, Argentina's pharmaceutical industry has the capacity to expand regional production and address vaccine access gaps. (Former Health Minister, 09–21–2021).

Technological and regulatory capacity-building allowed Insud and Richmond to expand their vaccine market horizons. Sinergium Biotech—also part of Insud Group, specialized in vaccine fill and finish—was selected by PAHO for the mRNA Technology Transfer Program in South Africa, gaining licenses and training to produce mRNA vaccines. This positioned Sinergium as a regional technology transfer hub, alongside Brazil's Fiocruz-BioManghinos (World Health Organization [WHO], 2023). The program, also requiring public involvement, also selected Argentina's ANLIS-Malbrán to produce vaccine lipids. Although a centennial public vaccine manufacturing and epidemiological reference, since the 2000s Malbrán had seen declining capacity due to policy shifts and industry concentration (Corvalán, 2017; Blume & Baylac-Paouly, 2021). After its role with Sputnik V, Richmond began building a new multi-platform biotechnology plant for vaccine and biological manufacturing, attracting funding through its elevated profile.

8.4.3 State Capacities Toward the "Argentine Vaccine"

Meanwhile, the public sector promoted STI projects to address the pandemic (Bortz & Gázquez, 2020). After COVID-19 was declared a national health emergency, the Ministry of Science, Technology, and Innovation (MINCyT), the National Science Council (CONICET), the Agency for R&D and Innovation (Agencia I + D + i), the MoH, and the Ministry of Industry created the Coronavirus Unit. This unprecedented coordination space aimed to accelerate health technology development by repurposing existing public sector R&D. In April 2020, the first competitive call (IP-COVID) was launched to support R&D projects on COVID-19 diagnostics, control, treatment, and monitoring. The design of proposal call and evaluation of over 900 projects were completed in record time, leveraging Agencia I + D + i's existing capacity. The project selection prioritized SARS-CoV-2 diagnostic kits, protective gear, and related technologies, excluding local vaccine development due to the country's lack of vaccine development experience and perceived infeasibility in an emergency.

Among the 125 IP-COVID funded projects was "Development of Tools to Prevent SARS-CoV-2 Infection," led by Dr. Juliana Cassataro, at the public Universidad Nacional de San Martín (UNSAM). By late 2020, her recombinant protein vaccine candidate ARVAC (Argentinian Vaccine) "Cecilia Grierson," had shown promising results. In November 2020, officials at the Agencia I + D + i connected the UNSAM group with the private sector, contacting various local biopharmaceutical laboratories with industrial capacity for recombinant proteins. A domestic biopharmaceutical firm, Laboratorio Pablo Cassará, accepted the challenge, leveraging its production capabilities, regulatory expertise, and prior vaccine experience.

Since December 2020, UNSAM and Cassará collaborated to scale up production and reformulate the adjuvant used in the vaccine prototype. The vaccine was designed to meet pediatric and maternal vaccination standards (Blanco, 2021; Pasquevich et al., 2023) and enable large-scale local production suited to Argentina's distribution infrastructure, requiring only standard refrigeration (2° to 8 °C) (Blanco, 2022; Peirano, 2023). ANMAT's prior regulatory experience with recombinant protein vaccines supported the aspiration of a swift approval. Building on these promising results, in April 2021, the Agencia I + D + i launched a new call for *in vivo* trials of Argentine vaccine candidates in preclinical phase, strengthening capacities (Agencia I+D+i, 2021).

ARVAC's Phase 1 clinical trials began in April 2022, funded with USD 7.5 million by Laboratorio Cassará (Noticias UNSAM, 2023, November 16). Phases 2/3 followed in January 2023, with USD eight million by the public STI sector (MINCYT, 06-03-2023). This direct, mission oriented funding to ARVAC was unprecedented for Agencia I + D + i, which typically relies on competitive grants, even for strategic projects. UNSAM assembled an administrative team to fast-track funding and manage resources for a clinical trial—unusual for a public institution. ANMAT also provided unprecedented support, supporting trial design, regulatory approval, and creating a new unit to support national innovation projects.

The final out of 2014 volunteers for ARVAC's Phase 3 was recruited on August 31, 2023 receiving ANMAT's approval on October 17, 2023 (Resolution 2023–8604) (Agencia I + D + i, 2023). This marked a national milestone: ARVAC became the first preventive vaccine for infectious diseases entirely designed and developed in Argentina, backed by unprecedented state coordination and investment. At USD 16 million, it was also one of the least expensive vaccines globally, compared to Comirnaty's USD 5.5 billion (Noticias UNSAM, 2023, November 16). However, the state has yet to purchase it, with mRNA vaccine supply purchased in late 2021 through a World Bank loan still remaining. Currently, the vaccine was released for commercialization in pharmacies and private vaccination centers (Vacunar, 2024).

Several state institutions built new supportive capabilities during this process. ANMAT was essential during the ARVAC project, supporting clinical trial design, and streamlining regulatory approval. Led by Dr. Cassataro at UNSAM, the project involved a 12-person research team with over 600 professionals from 24 public and private institutions, blending scientific, industrial, political, clinical, and organizational capacities (Noticias UNSAM, 2023, November 16). The initiative strengthened ties between the public STI sector and domestic biopharma, with officials promoting public–private partnerships, institutions funding and managing trials, and ANMAT building new capacities to assess locally developed vaccines. However, a political shift in late 2023 signaled a return to open market policies, not only failing to strengthen scientific, industrial, regulatory, coordination capabilities toward industrial development but purposefully dismantling them rather.

Key officials mobilized the imaginary of an active "present state" to reconfigure existing capacities and coordinate rapid, mission-driven responses (Mazzucato, 2023). Framed by a national sovereignty narrative, this discourse positioned the state as a catalyst for public–private collaboration and a driver of science and technology. It projected a "desirable future" rooted in self-reliance and sovereignty, aligning coalition actors around a redefined vision of autonomous healthcare access that allowed an unprecedented coordination, enabled by the state of emergency and even beyond.

> [After the regulatory approval of ARVAC] The *present state* and the political decision of a government to articulate with all the ministries. (Former Minister of Health) (Peirano, 2023)
>
> At a time when there are discussions about the importance of science in Argentina and about the role of the state, this development shows that sustained investment over the years in research, science, and technology leads to results like this. It is the *decision of a state* and a government to invest in science and technology and to have health sovereignty". (Former Minister of S&T, 2023)
>
> You need a *[state] decision* and funding to bring that [vaccine development] to the clinic and to the industry. (Biopharmaceutical industry CEO, *personal communication,* December 13, 2023).
>
> The pandemic has demonstrated the latent capabilities we had and the power of articulating public policies in these areas. (Former President R&D&I Agency) (Peirano, 2023).

The ARVAC development served as a demonstration effect by materializing the underlying promise of Argentine science to generate solutions to local problems through "useful" technologies (Herrera, 1973; Kreimer & Thomas, 2005; Zabala, 2009). The coalition that made this possible implied a delicate balance between the "static"—institutionalized capabilities—and the "dynamic" (Kattel et al., 2022). The latter refers to the capacities deployed by frontline managers in the government's CTI sector, who provided the ability to navigate established institutional frameworks, identify problems, and devise solutions based on their own and collective visions and ideas. However, in the current political context, in which the State and government are confronted involving institutional fragmentation and a cultural shift—toward individualism to the detriment of collective perspectives—many of the capacities that enabled coordination in the pandemic exceptional circumstances have been dismantled.

8.5 Discussion

State capacity involves not only mobilizing resources and institutions but using political agency to navigate diverse interests and ideologies, build consensus, and coordinate inter-organizational action around certain goals to foster social change. Analyzing how key state actors realign capacities toward shared goals—and how symbolic repertoires shape policy formation and legitimacy—is essential for understanding how a fragmented state advances driving change in a particular policy direction. This lens is vital to addressing today's complex challenges. The pandemic, as a state of exception, offers a unique opportunity to explore how crises can trigger adaptive capacity-building and redefine state roles.

Initially, key state actors identified vaccine access as a critical amid global demand and geopolitical tensions. Despite political and economic constraints, Argentina aligned—and partially built, not without delays—the capabilities needed to respond, from vaccine selection, to prioritizing knowledge building, and streamlining logistics for an unprecedented vaccination campaign. Delays with Pfizer were offset by acquiring Sputnik V, though not without controversy. ANMAT's technical expertise supported political decisions with scientific evidence. These efforts drew on the trajectory of the National Vaccination Program and the health ministry's frontline officials. Logistical capacities were repurposed to facilitate vaccine transport and distribution, recurring to the national airline, creating *ad-hoc* routes, expediting customs and ensuring swift coordination with subnational authorities.

During the crisis, scientists and STI policy makers aimed to legitimize the sector reorienting R&D capacities toward health technology, showcasing the relevance of its societal contribution. However, limited and outdated public manufacturing capacities hindered state-led vaccine production. To address these vulnerabilities, frontline policy makers played a key role in "patching up" state capabilities, critical during the immunization campaign (Prieto, 2023) by developing political and strategic capabilities. Despite constraints, public STI officials mobilized scientific and technological resources, partnering with the industry and aligning the Ministry of Health and regulatory agency to pursue a domestic vaccine. This was possible due to state-funded biomedical research and private manufacturing capabilities, supported by ANMAT's adaptive regulatory expertise.

The expertise of key officials and their technical teams was crucial for political agency—not only offering "know-how" and "know-what," but also "know-where": the ability to navigate institutional frameworks, align actors and resources, to identify problems and conceive solutions, and subtly shape policies through access to decision-making channels outlining the way forward. This ability is key to aligning actors and resources, as experts with access to decision-making channels can shape policies and subtly influence ideas, ideologies, and expectations. For instance, initial funding for a local vaccine was rejected due to skepticism rooted in past unfulfilled public R&D projects. Effective coordination between different types of institutionalized capacities, combined with "political entrepreneurs" in the mobilization of political-strategic visions—in co-constitution with sociotechnical imaginaries—for the creation of synergies between the public and productive sectors around shared means and ends, is a crucial condition for promoting highly complex and wide-ranging health projects.

While reliance on political figures enabled institutional flexibility and political maneuver in times of crisis, it also made the system vulnerable to political and economic shifts, hindering long-term knowledge retention and continuity that would survive cyclical governmental shifts. This poses a tension between the "know how" and "know where" embodied in state elites and the challenge of institutionalizing lasting public administration capabilities (or its actual feasibility).

The collective representation of the state and its role shaped coalition dynamics and resource alignment amid extreme uncertainty. The government's "present state" narrative—opposed to the "absent state", attributed to the opposition—aligned with broader sovereignty aspirations and served as a symbolic driver to mobilize capacities within fragmented structures toward a defined policy preference set. Beyond ensuring vaccine access, this narrative aimed to lay the groundwork to the aspiration of a fully national vaccine, strengthening long-term capabilities and public–private collaboration toward vaccine sovereignty and future health self-reliance. In yet another chapter of Argentina's recurring cyclic drama—where state and government collide amid political divides and re-foundational swings—most coordination structures built under the state of exception were dismantled by decree. While S&T is on the brink of collapse, capacities in some public sector institutions—universities, regulatory agencies—may endure. Yet what could have become institutionalized expertise to achieve ambitious development challenges now persists only in fragments, embodied in the individuals who once enabled coordination. As optimists, we hold on to hope—the quiet whisper that when the next storm comes, there will be time to rebuild.

References

Abrutzky, R., Bramuglia, C., & Godio, C. (2019). Institucionalización histórica de la salud como bien social en Argentina. *Sudamérica: Revista de Ciencias Sociales, 10*, 75–99.

Adler, E. (1987). *The power of ideology: The quest for technological autonomy in Argentina and Brazil.* University of California Press.

Agencia I+D+i. (2021, April 8). *Ensayos in vivo de vacunas argentinas COVID-19.* Retrieved September 9, 2024, from http://www.agencia.mincyt.gob.ar/frontend/agencia/convocatoria/449

Amengual, M., & Dargent, E. (2020). The social determinants of enforcement. *The politics of institutional weakness in Latin America*, 161–182.

Amoretti, L. (2023). La industria biofarmacéutica de Argentina y Brasil en el siglo XXI. *Ciencia, tecnología y política, 6*(10), 097.

Andrenacci, L. E. (2023). La gestión de la emergencia COVID-19 en Argentina (2020–2021). Un ejercicio de perspectiva artefactual y unas hipótesis para la investigación comparada. *Revista estudios de políticas públicas, 9*(2), 46–65.

Arce, H. E. (2010). El sistema de salud: De dónde viene y hacia dónde va. En: *El sistema de salud: de dónde viene y hacia dónde va.* Prometeo.

Arceo, E., & Basualdo, E. (2006). Los cambios en los sectores dominantes en América Latina bajo el Neoliberalismo. *Neoliberalismo y sectores dominantes. Tendencias globales y experiencias nacionales*, 15–26.

Azpiazu, D. (1999). *Las renegociaciones contractuales en los servicios públicos privatizados:= seguridad jurídica o preservación de ventas de privilegio?*

Balajewder, F., Sampson, S., & Stratton, T. (March, 2021). Lessons for industrial policy from development of the Oxford/AstraZeneca Covid-19 vaccine. *Industrial Strategy Council, Research Paper.*

Belló, M., & Becerril-Montekio, V. M. (2011). Sistema de salud de Argentina. *Salud Pública de México, 53*(2), 96–109.

Besley, T. (2006). *Principled agents?: The political economy of good government.* Oxford University Press.

Blanco, D. (2020, December 15). *Las bondades científicas de la vacuna de Pfizer-Biontech que lidera planes de vacunación del mundo: ¿Por qué no la tenemos?* Retrieved December 28, from en: https://www.infobae.com/salud/2020/12/16/las-bondades-cientificas-de-la-vacun-de-pfizer-biontech-que-lidera-los-planes-devacunacion-del-mundo-por-que-no-la-tenemos

Blanco, D. (2021, December 13). *Vacuna argentina ARVAC-Cecilia Grierson contra el COVID-19: Por qué emerge como la más prometedora contra Ómicron y nuevas variantes*. Retrieved September 9, 2024, from https://www.infobae.com/america/ciencia-america/2021/12/13/vacuna-argentina-arvac-cecilia-grierson-contra-el-covid-19-por-que-emerge-como-la-mas-prometedora-contra-omicron-y-nuevas-variantes

Blanco, D. (2022, March 30). *La vacuna argentina ARVAC Cecilia Grierson contra COVID vista en claves fundamentales*. Retrieved December 28, 2023, from https://www.infobae.com/salud/ciencia/2022/03/30/la-vacuna-argentina-arvac-cecilia-grierson-contra-covid-vista-en-tres-claves-fundamentales

Blinder, D., Zubeldía, L., & Surtayeva, S. (2021). Covid-19 and semi-periphery. *Journal of World-Systems Research, 27*(2).

Blofield, M., Pribble, J., & Giambruno, C. (2023). *The politics of social protection during times of crisis*. Cambridge University Press.

Blume, S., & Baylac-Paouly, B. (Eds.). (2021). *Immunization and states: The politics of making vaccines*. Routledge.

Boletín Oficial. Aislamiento Social, Preventivo y Obligatorio. 19 marzo 2020. Retrieved December 28, 2023, from https://www.boletinoficial.gob.ar/detalleAviso/primera/227042/20200320

Bortz, G. M., & Gázquez, A. (2020). Políticas CTI en Argentina durante la pandemia: ¿Oportunidad para nuevas redes participativas en I+D+i? Debates sobre Innovación, 5(1), 16–23. Universidad Autónoma Metropolitana.

Bortz, G., & Sanmartin, M. C. (2023). Vacunas y vacunaciones: Capacidades, políticas y visiones sobre el Estado frente al COVID-19 en Argentina. *Revista Iberoamericana de Ciencia, Tecnología y Sociedad-CTS*. Retrieved from https://ojs.revistacts.net/index.php/CTS/article/view/509

Bracco, O. N., & Porta Fernández, P. (2022). Clivajes políticos en tiempos de pandemia: Una aproximación a las representaciones de la ciudadanía en Argentina (2020–2022). *Sociohistórica, 50*, 170–170.

Callon, M. (1990). Techno-economic networks and irreversibility. *The Sociological Review, 38*(S1), 132–161. https://doi.org/10.1111/j.1467-954X.1990.tb03351.x

Caravaca, J., & Daniel, C. (2023). *Afrontar lo inesperado: El Estado argentino ante la crisis global del COVID-19*. Editorial Biblos.

Charmaz, K. (2016). Shifting the grounds: Constructivist grounded theory methods. In Developing grounded theory (pp. 127–193). Routledge.

CILFA. (2021, March). *La industria farmacéutica argentina: Su carácter estratégico y perspectivas* (1), *Cámara Industrial de Laboratorios Farmacéuticos Argentinos*. https://cilfa.org.ar/wp1/wp-content/uploads/2021/07/Escenario-y-Perspectivas-de-la-Industria-Farmaceutica-Argentina-2021.pdf

Comisión Técnica Asesora de Salud. (2020). *COVID-19: Acceso a medicamentos y vacunas*. Retrieved Month Date, Year, from https://www.argentina.gob.ar/noticias/covid-19-acceso-medicamentos-y-

Corrales, J. (2018). *Fixing democracy: Why constitutional change often fails to enhance democracy in Latin America*. Oxford University Press.

Correa, J., De la Puente, C., Picasso, R., & Silvestrini, C. (2023). *Patentamiento de anticuerpos monoclonales: El caso de Argentina*. 186, Econstor.

Corvalán, D. (2017). Des-aprendizaje y pérdida de capacidades locales: El calendario nacional de vacunación en Argentina. *Ciencia, docencia y tecnología, 54*, 1–37.

David, P. A. (1994). Why are institutions the 'carriers of history'?: Path dependence and the evolution of conventions, organizations and institutions. *Structural Change and Economic Dynamics, 5*(2), 205–220.

Demonte, F., Bruno, D. P., Lozano, L. S., Mena, M. F., & Pereira, A. M. (2024). Conversación pública sobre vacunas en la pandemia de covid-19 en Argentina, 2021–2022. *Salud colectiva, 20*, 4580.

Dezalay, Y., & Garth, B. G. (Eds.). (2002). *Global prescriptions: The production, exportation, and importation of a new legal orthodoxy*. University of Michigan Press.

Diputados Argentina. (2021, February 2). *Visita del Ministro de Salud, Dr. Ginés Gonzales García y su equipo*. Comisión Permanente de Acción Social y Salud Pública. Retrieved March 11, 2025, from https://www.hcdn.gob.ar/comisiones/permanentes/casyspublica/reuniones/vts/vtcom.html?id=7880

Estévez, A. M. (2001). *La reforma managerialista del Estado: Nueva gerencia pública, calidad total y tecnocracia*. Buenos Aires; Ediciones Cooperativas.

Ezrahi, Y. (1990). *The descent of Icarus: Science and the transformation of contemporary democracy*. Harvard University Press.

Fajnzylber, F. (1998). *Industrialización en América Latina: de la "caja negra" al "casillero vacío"*. Selección.

Fukuyama, F. (2013). What is governance? *Governance, 26*(3), 347–368.

Fundación Bunge y Born. (2021). *Índice de confianza y Acceso a Vacunas 2020.02 febrero*.

Geddes, B. (1994). Challenging the conventional wisdom. *Journal of Democracy, 5*(4), 104–118.

Giraudo, M. E., & Grugel, J. (2022). Imaginaries of soy and the costs of commodity-led development: Reflections from Argentina. *Development and Change, 53*(4), 796–826.

Gollan, D., Kreplak, N., & Garcia, E. (2021). *La salud sí tiene precio: Medicamentos, hospitales, pandemias y la necesidad de repensar el sistema sanitario*. Siglo XXI Editores.

Gutman, G. E. (2018). Biotecnología en salud humana: Experiencias en países pioneros países de ingreso tardío. *Centro de Estudios Urbanos y Regionales*, 109–140.

Gutman, G., & Lavarello, P. (2016). *Política industrial en el sector biofarmacéutico en la Argentina durante los años 2000*. CEPAL.

Hameiri, S. (2007). Failed states or a failed paradigm? State capacity and the limits of institutionalism. *Journal of International Relations and Development, 10*, 122–149.

Heredia, M. (2022). *Qué pudo y qué no pudo el Estado: Frente a la emergencia de covid-19 y después*. Siglo XXI Editores.

Herrera, A. O. (1973). Los determinantes sociales de la política científica en América Latina: Política científica explícita y política científica implícita. *Desarrollo Económico*, 113–134.

Infobae. (2020a, November 5). *Alberto Fernández hablará hoy con Vladimir Putin por la compra que la Argentina hará de la vacuna rusa contra el coronavirus*. Retrieved September 9, 2024, from https://www.infobae.com/politica/2020/11/05/alberto-fernandez-hablara-manana-con-vladimir-putin-por-la-compra-que-la-argentina-hara-de-la-vacuna-rusa-contra-el-coronavirus

Infobae. (2020b, August 12). *Quién es quién en la fabricación de la vacuna del COVID-19 en la Argentina*. Retrieved December 28, 2023, from https://www.infobae.com/economia/2020/08/13/quien-es-quien-en-la-fabricacion-de-la-vacuna-del-covid-19-enlaargentina/#:~:text=Seg%C3%BAn%20las%20palabras%20de%20Alberto,si%20se%20utilizaban%20otras%20opciones

Infobae. (2021, February 26). *Qué implica que la vacuna Sputnik V se produzca en la Argentina*. Retrieved September 9, 2024, from https://www.infobae.com/salud/2021/02/26/que-implica-que-la-vacuna-sputnik-v-se-produzca-en-la-argentina

Jasanoff, S. (2004). The idiom of co-production. In Editor(s) Name(s), *States of knowledge* (pp. 1–12). Routledge.

Jasanoff, S., & Kim, S. H. (Eds.). (2019). *Dreamscapes of modernity: Sociotechnical imaginaries and the fabrication of power*. University of Chicago Press.

Joerges, B. (1999). Do politics have artefacts? *Social Studies of Science, 29*(3), 411–431.

Joly, P. B. (2010). On the economics of techno-scientific promises. *Débordements. Mélanges offerts à Michel Callon*, 203–222.

Kattel, R., Drechsler, W., & Karo, E. (2022). *How to make an entrepreneurial state: Why innovation needs bureaucracy*. Yale University Press.

Kreimer, P. (2010). *Ciencia y periferia. Nacimiento, muerte y resurrección de la biología molecular en la Argentina. Aspectos sociales, políticos y cognitivos*. Eudeba.

Kreimer, P., & Thomas, H. (2005). What is CANA-AKNA? Social Utility of Scientific and Technological Knowledge: Challenges for Latin American Research Centers. *Development Through Knowledge*, 59–82.

La Nación. (2021, June 8). *Solo "envasan" vacunas: La decepción de científicos de Richmond ante las críticas*. Retrieved September 8, 2024, from https://www.lanacion.com.ar/sociedad/solo-envasan-vacunas-la-tristeza-de-cientificos-de-richmond-ante-las-criticas-nid08062021

La Serna, C. (2013). Imaginarios y materialidades en la transformación del Estado en la Argentina de la última década. *Revista de ciencias sociales, 5*(23).

Lavarello, P. J., Gutman, G., & Pita, J. J. (2023). Biosimilars and Heterogeneous Technological Trajectories in the Argentine Biopharmaceutical Industry. *Journal of Law, Medicine & Ethics, 51*(S1), 116–125.

Lerner, E. (1988). *Gasto público, rol del Estado y regímenes políticos*. Doctoral Dissertation, Facultad de Ciencias Económicas, Universidad de Buenos Aires.

Levitsky, S., & Murillo, M. V. (2005). *Argentine democracy: The politics of institutional weakness*. Penn State Press.

Lundvall, B. Ä., & Johnson, B. (1994). The learning economy. *Journal of Industry Studies, 1*(2), 23–42.

Maceira, D. (2020). Caracterización del sistema de salud argentino. Debate en el contexto Latinoamericano. *Revista Estado y Políticas Públicas, 14*, 155–179. Retrieved from http://repositorio.cedes.org/handle/123456789/4536

Madoery, O. (2005). *La "primera generación" de políticas locales de desarrollo en Argentina: Contexto, características y desafíos. Argentina*. Centro de Estudios Desarrollo y Territorio (CEDeT).

Mann, M. (1984). The autonomous power of the state: Its origins, mechanisms and results. *European Journal of Sociology/Archives Européennes de Sociologie, 25*(2), 185–213.

Marin, G. H. (2021). El sistema de salud argentino: Un análisis a partir del acceso a los medicamentos. *Ciência e Saúde Coletiva, 26*, 5453–5462.

Mazzucato, M. (2011). The entrepreneurial state. *Soundings, 49*(49), 131–142.

Mazzucato, M. (2018). Mission-oriented innovation policies: Challenges and opportunities. *Industrial and Corporate Change, 27*(5), 803–815.

Mazzucato, M. (2023). Financing the Sustainable Development Goals through mission-oriented development banks. *UN DESA Policy Brief Special issue*. UN Department of Economic and Social Affairs and UCL Institute for Innovation and Public Purpose. New York, USA.

Merino, M. A. G. (2004). *América Latina en el siglo XXI: Hacia una nueva matriz sociopolítica*. Lom Ediciones.

Migdal, J. S. (1988). *Strong societies and weak states: State-society relations and state capabilities in the Third World*. Princeton University Press.

Migdal, J. S. (2004). State building and the non-nation-state. *Journal of International Affairs, 58*, 17–46.

MoH. (2020, December 24). *Llegaron al país las primeras vacunas SPUTNIK*. Retrieved September 9, 2024, from https://www.argentina.gob.ar/noticias/llegaron-al-pais-las-primerasvacunassputnikv#:~:text=Hoy%20empezamos%20un%20nuevo%20caminopalabras%20de%20agradecimiento%20para%20ellos.%E2%80%9D

MoH. (2023, May 31). *Se creó la Unidad para la Gestión Integral del Riesgo en Salud*. Retrieved September 9, 2024, from https://www.argentina.gob.ar/noticias/se-creo-la-unidad-para-la-gestion-integral-del-riesgo-en-salud

MoH. (2024, September 8). *Administración Nacional de Medicamentos, Alimentos y Tecnología Médica*. Retrieved September 8, 2022, from https://www.argentina.gob.ar/anmat/gestion-de-calidad/que-es-la-anmat

Naciones Unidas. (2021, Septemebr 23). *Análisis conjunto del Sistema de Naciones Unidas 2021: Los efectos de la pandemia por COVID-19 en la Argentina*. United Nations. Retrieved

September 9, 2024, from https://argentina.un.org/es/145708-an%C3%A1lisis-conjunto-del-sistema-de-naciones-unidas-2021-los-efectos-de-la-pandemia-por-covid

Naspleda, F. D. (2023). Transformación en la industria farmacéutica argentina: Del liderazgo de las empresas internacionales Big Pharma al dominio de las corporaciones locales de genéricos de marca (2003–2018). *Anuario Centro de Estudios Económicos de la Empresa y el Desarrollo, 19*, 169–212.

Neaera Abers, R., Rossi, F. M., & von Bülow, M. (2021). state–society relations in uncertain times: Social movement strategies, ideational contestation and the pandemic in Brazil and Argentina. *International Political Science Review, 42*(3), 333–349. https://doi.org/10.1177/0192512121993713

Nochteff, H. (2001). *La experiencia argentina de los 90 desde el enfoque de la competitividad sistémica*. FLACSO-Argentina.

Noticias UNSAM. (2023, November 16). *ARVAC, la clave de ingreso al mundo biofarma*. Retrieved September 9, 2024, from https://noticias.unsam.edu.ar/2023/11/15/arvac-la-clave-de-ingreso-al-mundo-biofarma/

Olin, I. (2018). La incorporación de la vacuna contra varicela al Calendario Nacional de Vacunación en Argentina: ≚Cómo se llegó a esta política pública?. *Independent Study Project (ISP) Collection*. Retrieved from https://digitalcollections.sit.edu/isp_collection/2947

Ottervik, M. (2013). *Conceptualizing and measuring state capacity* (QoG Working Paper 2013–20). Gothenburg: The Quality of Government Institute, University of Gothenburg.

Pasquale, C. A., et al. (2022). Immunogenicity and reactogenicity of heterologous immunization against SARS CoV-2 using Sputnik V, ChAdOx1-S, BBIBP-CorV, Ad5-nCoV, and mRNA-1273. *Cell Reports Medicine, 3*(8).

Pasquevich, K. A., Coria, L. M., Ceballos, A., Mazzitelli, B., Rodriguez, J. M., Demaría, A., & Cassataro, J. (2023). Safety and immunogenicity of a SARS-CoV-2 Gamma variant RBD-based protein adjuvanted vaccine used as booster in healthy adults. *Nature Communications, 14*(1), 4551.

Peirano, F. (2023, October 21). *La Argentina que funciona y su primera vacuna*. Infobae. Retrieved September 9, 2024, from https://www.infobae.com/opinion/2023/10/21/la-argentina-que-funciona-y-su-primera-vacuna

Perissinotto, R. M. (2021). Ideas, burocracia e industrialización en Argentina y Brasil (1930–1966). *Lenguaje Claro Editora*.

Prieto, J. D. (2023). The distributive politics of social assistance targeting: Evidence from COVID-19 relief in Colombia. *Social Policy & Administration, 57*(5), 744–759.

Romero, L. A. (2016). *Entre pipetas, bisturíes y pacientes: La investigación clínica en la*.

Rosso, G. (2023). Los imaginarios de la "nueva política" en Argentina: Un estudio de la red simbólica de PRO-Cambiemos (2015–2017). *Imagonautas, 12*(17), 241–263.

Rothstein, B. (2011). *The quality of government: Corruption, social trust, and inequality in international perspective*. University of Chicago Press.

Rovere, M. (2004). *La salud en la Argentina: Alianzas y conflictos en la construcción de un sistema injusto*. Revista electrónica La Esquina del Sur.

Rudek, T. J. (2022). Capturing the invisible. Sociotechnical imaginaries of energy. The critical overview. *Science and Public Policy, 49*(2), 219–245.

Sanmartin, M. C. (2023). Propiedad intelectual y salud pública en países en desarrollo: Vino viejo en odres nuevos. *Hipertextos, 11*(19), 067–067.

Sanmartin, M. C., & Bortz, G. (2024). Coaliciones de producción de vacunas COVID-19. Una mirada desde América Latina. *Revista Brasileña de Innovación, 23*, e024003.

Santos, G., & Thomas, H. (2018). Producción pública de medicamentos: Desafíos para una política estratégica en materia de salud. *Ciencia, tecnología y política, 1*(1), 007–007.

Schot, J., & Steinmueller, W. E. (2018). Three frames for innovation policy: R&D, systems of innovation and transformative change. *Research Policy, 47*(9), 1554–1567.

Skocpol, T. (1979). state and revolution: Old regimes and revolutionary crises in France, Russia, and China. *Theory and Society, 7*, 7–95.

Smink, V. (2021, April 29). *Vacunas contra la covid-19: qué pasó con los millones de dosis de AstraZeneca que México y Argentina prometieron producir en América Latina*. BBC News. Retrieved September 9, 2024, from https://www.bbc.com/mundo/noticias-america-latina-56923216

Spinelli, H. (2010). Las dimensiones del campo de la salud en Argentina. *Salud Colectiva, 6*, 275–293.

Stubrin, L. (2022). Un análisis del crecimiento de la actividad biotecnológica en la Argentina en clave sistémica (1982–2022). *Desarrollo económico, 62*(236), 50–78.

Thomas, S. J., Moreira, E. D., Jr., Kitchin, N., Jansen, K. U., et al. (2021). Safety and efficacy of the BNT162b2 mRNA Covid-19 vaccine through 6 months. *New England Journal of Medicine, 385*(19), 1761–1773.

Tilly, C. (1991). Domination, resistance, compliance... discourse. *Eastern Sociological Society, 6*, 593–602.

Tommasi, M., & Spiller, P. (2007). The institutional foundations of public policy in Argentina. Un ejercicio de perspectiva artefactual y unas hipótesis para la investigación comparada. In: *Índice de Confianza en el Gobierno*. Universidad Torcuato Di Tella, Abril 2020 y 2021.

Vacunar. (2024, May 10). *Vacuna ARVAC contra el COVID-19*. Retrieved September 9, 2024, from https://vacunar.com.ar/vacuna-arvac-contra-covid-19

Vanderslott, S., Emary, K., te Water Naude, R., English, M., Thomas, T., Patrick-Smith, M., et al. (2021). Vaccine nationalism and internationalism: Perspectives of COVID-19 vaccine trial participants in the United Kingdom. *BMJ Global Health, 6*(10), e006305.

Vilas, C. M. (1997). De ambulancias, bomberos y policías: La política social del neoliberalismo. *Desarrollo económico, 36*, 931–952.

Weiss, L., & Thurbon, E. (2022). Explaining divergent national responses to Covid-19: An enhanced state capacity framework. *New Political Economy, 27*(4), 697–712.

Winner, L. (1993). Social constructivism: Opening the black box and finding it empty. *Science as Culture, 3*(3), 427–452.

World Health Organization. (2023, June). *The mRNA vaccine technology transfer hub*. Retrieved September 9, 2024, from https://www.who.int/initiatives/the-mrna-vaccine-technology-transfer-hub

Zabala, J. P. (2009). Historia de la enfermedad de Chagas en Argentina: Evolución conceptual, institucional y política. *História, Ciências, Saúde-Manguinhos, 16*, 57–74.

Zhang, A. Z. (2021). Analysis of Pfizer Inc. under COVID-19. *Academic Journal of Business & Management, 3*(4), 15–17.

Chapter 9
Conclusion

Isamu Okada and Takahiro Miyachi

9.1 Introduction

The COVID-19 pandemic is not the first and is unlikely to be the last pandemic in human history. Therefore, we must draw lessons from the latest pandemic and prepare well to save lives and other negative consequences in the future. This book addresses cross-national patterns in the responses of Latin American states and society to the pandemic.

In particular, this book has addressed the following three questions.

- What do state strengths and weaknesses explain about the responses and outcomes to the COVID-19 pandemic?
- What solutions were practically available when state capacity was weak or limited?
- What does the COVID-19 pandemic update with the meaning of state capacity?

The first question takes state capacity as an independent variable that potentially explains outcomes under the COVID-19 pandemic. As argued in Chap. 1, state capacity has not been properly considered or used to explain the phenomena associated with the pandemic, particularly in Latin America. Yet, looking beyond the region, state capacity revolves around scholarly debates worldwide and is considered vital in explaining less severe consequences in other regions. This scant attention in Latin America is also a surprise given the presence of serial works contributing to theoretical sophistication from the inter- and intra-regional comparisons (Kurtz, 2013; Saylor, 2014; Soifer, 2015). Chapters 2–5 of this collective volume address this gap through comparative approaches.

I. Okada (✉) · T. Miyachi
Nagoya University, The University of Tokyo, Nagoya, Tokyo, Japan
e-mail: okada.isamu.w8@f.mail.nagoya-u.ac.jp

I. Okada (ed.), *COVID-19 and State Capacity in Latin America*, Latin American Societies, https://doi.org/10.1007/978-3-032-15572-6_9

The second question looks beyond the weak state capacity in Latin America. Scholarly views coincide that Latin America has been plagued with state weaknesses rather than strengths (Brinks et al., 2020; Helmke & Levitsky, 2004; Yashar, 2018). That, however, has also brought attention to societal engagements with weak state presence. Institutional weaknesses can be derived and complemented by the creative use of existing institutions or collaborative governance and co-production between state and societal actors. Chapters 6–8 deal with the puzzle and draw lessons on state weaknesses.

Meanwhile, the third question revisits the meaning of state capacity from the case of the COVID-19 pandemic. State capacity is a multifaceted concept, and what capacity matters when facing a specific kind of crisis is of high interest. Health infrastructure, policy coordination, and resource mobilization are basic capacities essential to deliver and expand urgent responses. Hard lockdowns require coercive capacity to ensure compliance. Voluntary behavioral changes necessitate trust and communication skills. State capacity is primarily attached to the state, but it also encompasses networks and partnerships with societal actors.

The following sections summarize key takeaways for each of the three questions. Table 9.1 summarizes key takeaways from our findings, which will be explained in more detail in the following sections.

Table 9.1 Key takeaways

Q1 What do state strengths and weaknesses explain about the responses and outcomes to the COVID-19 pandemic?	
1	State capacity variations have explanatory power on policy variation and consequences.
2	Latin American states were not strong or present enough in general.
3	State capacity's effect varied according to the capacity dimension and outcomes.
Q2 What solutions were practically available when state capacity was weak or limited?	
4	Facing weak state capacity, Latin American states used several practical solutions.
5	State-society collaboration was present at some cases but absent in many instances.
Q3 What does the COVID-19 pandemic update with the meaning of state capacity?	
6	State capacity is multidimensional, including administrative capacity, effective communication and trust-building with citizens, financial investment in health infrastructure and human resources, etc.
7	The state is non-unitary and engages in collaborative governance with a variety of public and private actors.
8	State capacity is recognized as a long-term factor. Short-term responses through emulation and state-society collaboration were observed, but whether those evolve into institutional updates is a topic of future studies.

Source: Author

9.2 What Do State Strengths and Weaknesses Explain About the Responses and Outcomes to the COVID-19 Pandemic?

This volume provides several lessons regarding the first question. First, state capacity variations have explanatory power on policy variations and consequences. Second, the regional states were not strong or present in general when they were needed. Third, the effects of state capacity vary according to the capacity and outcomes we look at. We discuss each point in turn.

As the first lesson, the chapters that adopt a comparative perspective on the direct provision of public goods confirm that countries with higher state capacity are more likely to implement measures appropriately and sufficiently, leading to better protection of their societies. Chapter 2 (Bizberg and Jiménez Hernández) demonstrates that countries with weak medical infrastructure, such as Bolivia, Ecuador, and Peru, experienced high excess mortality rates. In contrast, the opposite of the spectrum, such as Argentina, Brazil, Costa Rica, and Uruguay, reported low excess deaths. Isolating Brazil and Mexico as exceptions, where political agencies disturbed canonical non-pharmaceutical measures, other regional peers show a comparative trend echoing what previous intra-regional rankings have presupposed.

Chapter 3 (Okada) further develops this standpoint with deeper and more careful scrutiny of state capacity measurement. While official indicators reported by international organizations tend to suffer a reporting bias endogenous to the very state's capacity to collect accurate information—hence making true value ambiguous—this chapter approaches what people experienced and informed from a daily survey. Remarkably, the survey-based test capacity gap, by and large, overlaps general state capacity indicators like Government Effectiveness by the World Bank's Worldwide Governance Indicator (WGI) and Fragility Index. Moreover, the test capacity gap provides a good prediction of the COVID-19 case fatality rate, reconfirming the finding of Chap. 2: state capacity does explain key outcomes during the pandemic. These findings corroborate the explanatory advantage of state capacity, an argument similar to previous studies (Alfano & Ercolano, 2022; Bosancianu et al., 2020; Gisselquist & Vaccaro, 2023; Serikbayeva et al., 2021) but more carefully and directly applied in the Latin American context.

Despite the fact that state capacity improves health outcomes during the pandemic, the second lesson informs that Latin American states were often not very effective or absent when it was needed. This becomes more obvious in how citizens perceive and react to the government's actions. Chapter 4 (Miyachi) analyzes central government announcements on mask-wearing and finds that effective messaging was not necessarily tied to high state capacity. In rare cases, low state capacity even facilitated compliance. This suggests that citizens followed government announcements not because of trust in their government's capacity but because they saw them as warnings about the severity of the pandemic and took independent action to protect themselves.

Another evidence of the state's absence is manifested in Chap. 7 (Bianchi, Coda, and Santamarina), which highlights the chronic shortage of government resources in Latin American countries that leads politicians to adopt a bleak outlook on pandemic management. As the same chapter emphasizes, collaborative governance between the state and societal actors was usually ad hoc and short-lived, seldom institutionalized during the pandemic. This was more so for the marginalized people in the region, who had to stand and help each other among themselves.

Chapter 8 (Sanmartín and Bortz), however, submits a counterargument to this state absence theorem. According to the authors, "the absent state" and "the neoliberal ghost" are the discussions of the 1990s, and the situation changed to a stronger or more efficient state intervention from the 2000s. Unsure if vaccine production is distinctive as a policy issue, which we will discuss later, but they add more nuance to the whole debate by highlighting the accumulation of institutional capacity and public–private co-production that eventually enabled one of the least expensive vaccines made in Argentina.

The third lesson is related to the variation in the effect of state capacity. Following the research orientation outlined in Chap. 1 (Okada), which emphasizes the importance of distinguishing capacity across different sectors and concrete policy targets, the chapters in this collection closely address various issues, from preventing infection and excess deaths (Chaps. 2, 3, and 5), coronavirus testing (Chap. 3), mask-wearing (Chap. 4), urgent issuance of measures (Chap. 6), support to the subsistence of marginalized people (Chap. 7), and vaccine manufacturing (Chap. 8).

These different policy targets are subject to different state capacity dimensions, of course, such that preventing infection and mortality is related to health infrastructure, which is broader than the specific capacity associated with testing expansion and vaccine development. This variation in mechanism and associated capacity dimension naturally leads to uneven causal linkages by policy target.

A careful review of our chapters concludes that some policy targets and associated capacity dimensions show a more significant impact on outcomes than others. As Chaps. 2 and 3 demonstrate, major health outcomes such as excess mortality and case fatality rates are closely related to government effectiveness and the actual provision of health services (how many tests are eventually supplied). This causal linkage is less apparent for mask-wearing, as reported in Chap. 4, which depends on communication, perception, and behavioral change. As other chapters repeatedly suggest, Latin American states are, by and large, distrusted.

A further interesting contrast is exhibited in the state-society collaborations. When the policy target was the protection of marginalized populations, states were widely absent (Chap. 7). Conversely, in vaccine production (Chap. 8), resources and collaboration converged between the state and the public sector. This contrast poses questions about collaborative governance, regarding who and for what purpose the collaboration occurs. Beyond collaborative governance, several studies have highlighted that state-building and policymaking in Latin America have sometimes been through the coalition of political and economic elites at distinctive subnational territories (Eaton, 2017; Saylor, 2014). This suggests that collaborations are articulated according to resources, power, and capacities each actor possesses; thus, more collaborations tend to happen among elites who mobilize expertise and resources than ordinary citizens.

Summing up the arguments, state capacity has explanatory power for health outcomes but remains largely unsatisfactory and varies across policy targets and capacity dimensions. It should be emphasized that these findings were made possible by this volume's commitment to methodological plurality, which is an essential feature for addressing the complexity of the COVID-19 pandemic. Rather than assuming a straightforward correlation between state capacity and policy effectiveness, we recognized that such relationships are often mediated by contextual, sectoral, and political variables. Accordingly, each chapter employed methodological approaches best suited to its specific research question and empirical setting, from computational text analysis and survey-based indicators to institutional process tracing and qualitative policy evaluation. This pluralistic approach was not incidental but necessary: to question the assumption that higher state capacity uniformly leads to more effective pandemic responses, we had to move beyond methodological simplism and adopt analytical tools tailored to the diversity of policy domains and real-world conditions under examination.

These findings derive from the book's regional focus on Latin America, which enabled a nuanced and context-sensitive exploration of how state capacity relates to policy variety and outcomes within a culturally similar regional setting. The chapters interrogate variations among countries that share historical legacies, institutional features, and normative expectations. Even in those employing quantitative techniques, the authors incorporate contextual knowledge to interpret findings meaningfully, thereby avoiding the pitfalls of decontextualized statistical generalization. Drawing on fine-grained data, case-specific observations, and sectoral disaggregation, this volume traces the mechanisms through which state capacity shapes, and at times fails to shape, concrete policy responses during the pandemic. The result is neither a simplistic assertion that "more capacity equals better outcomes" nor a claim that Latin America exhibits a peculiar pattern of connection between state capacity and policy variety. Instead, the book offers a layered understanding of how different capacities interact with specific policy demands under real-world constraints, and invites scholars working on other regions to adopt a similarly context-sensitive perspective when examining the complex manifestations of state capacity in public policy.

9.3 What Solutions Were Practically Available When State Capacity Was Weak or Limited?

The second question addressed in this book concerns what solutions were available when state capacity was weak or limited during the COVID-19 pandemic. There are many reasons for weak or limited state capacity in Latin America. The first and foremost is the structural constraints, which, by their very structural nature, are not easily resolved in the short term. Such structural constraints range from lack of sufficient revenue for the state and income for citizens to historically rooted social mistrust of public institutions and entrenched social discriminations, including gender-based ones, which all take a long time to overcome. Compared to Germany and Asian countries, whose pandemic responses were highly evaluated in Chap. 2, Latin American countries face an inherently disadvantageous starting position.

Facing weak state capacity, Latin American states used several practical solutions. The chapters in this collection highlight the emulations of other states and collaborations with societal actors.

Chapter 6 (Kikuchi) employs computational text analysis to measure the similarity of executive orders issued in the early stages of the pandemic. The study reveals a correlation between low administrative capacity and the tendency to mimic other countries' policies. The author tentatively interprets this as evidence that governments with low administrative capacity apparently adopted easily implementable policies. In addition to Chap. 6, other chapters in this book also discuss policy imitations. Imitation itself is not inherently negative; rather, it represents knowledge-sharing that expands a country's policy repertoire. However, as exemplified by the mechanical enforcement of mask-wearing mandates in Chap. 4, policies that ignore social context do not lead to effective outcomes. Reflecting on the political and social ramifications of policies is a fundamental task for politicians and bureaucrats to avoid investing effort in ineffective measures.

This volume also presents collaborative cases between governmental and non-governmental actors. While Chap. 7 generally underscores the absence of government involvement in collaborative governance across Latin America, it also highlights instances where governments actively engaged in pandemic responses. The diffusion of Centinela Renca, a COVID-19 tracking software in Chile, resulted from a collaboration between local governments and civil society actors, both national and international, as well as the decision of adjacent governments to adopt the software after observing its effectiveness. Additionally, Chap. 8 (Sanmartín and Bortz) extends the analysis of agency by tracing the process through which the Argentine government established its vaccine supply policy. Drawing on Science and Technology Studies (STS), the authors describe policymaking as a network of human and non-human interactions, moving away from anthropocentric approaches common in political process analysis. The study demonstrates how objects such as vaccines and digital platforms, as well as ideological imaginaries like the "present state" as an antithesis to neoliberalism, influenced policymakers' decision-making.[1]

Tackling weak state capacity in the short run, however, was sometimes hampered by political demotivation. Chapters 2 and 7 indicate that democratic regimes, compounded by the aforementioned historical structures, can dissuade politicians from implementing anti-pandemic policies. As discussed in Chap. 2, the hesitance of

[1] Chapter 7, although the authors do not explicitly mention it, also refers to non-human agencies, such as debit cards, which inspired the Argentine municipality to organize equitable community kitchens, and biosecurity measures that enabled the market in El Alto, Bolivia, to remain open during the pandemic.

populist presidents to proactively address COVID-19 stems from their reliance on public popularity, making it difficult for them to implement unpopular policies such as movement restrictions that would slow down economic activities. This argument aligns with Chap. 7's discussion of electoral pressures as an impediment to collaborative governance.

Similarly, other structural factors also limited policymakers and citizens from exercising agency for collaborations. Chapter 7 explains the general absence of collaborative governance in Latin American countries as a consequence of a historical structure. The same chapter also highlights how societal structures can obstruct interest representation and desirable policy choices. Its case study on Bolivia reveals that, despite the fact that the majority of the informal sector workforce is female, most representatives of informal labor organizations in discussing government policies were male, reflecting Bolivian society's biased gender structure. Countries in the so-called Global South, including those in Latin America, have suffered from a lack of public resources, chronic corruption, and polarized political competition. All these factors serve as barriers to cooperation between actors inside and outside governments in pursuing the public good.

9.4 What Does the COVID-19 Pandemic Update with the Meaning of State Capacity?

The third question asks what, in the end, we learn about state capacity from the COVID-19 pandemic. The answer to this question has already been discussed to some extent in the previous sections. In principle, state capacity is multidimensional and varies in impact across capacity dimensions. State capacity has a specific meaning in health sector, and particularly the responses to the pandemic, thus our understanding will remain limited if we rely solely on generic indicators.

Section 9.2 suggests that state capacity has multiple dimensions that connect them to different policy targets. In the long run, the state is expected to build a robust health infrastructure spread across territories within a country. In the short run, it must strengthen its administrative capacity to supply services swiftly. In the meantime, the state should also win citizens' trust and self-compliance, which Latin American states have substantive challenges. Some of these dimensions require substantive financial investment over time, while others necessitate effective human resource management through an appropriate organizational structure. In general, some countries are considered advanced in most of the dimensions, while others lag behind. Such an intra-regional ranking has been persistent for decades. State capacity gaps shaped and maintained over Latin American history are manifested in the capacity gaps in the state responses to the pandemic.

State capacity as a long-time factor holds true to some extent, but the capacity is possibly reshaped and rebuilt at a critical moment. Some findings suggest that state capacity remains mostly stable over time in some sense. Analysis in Chap. 3 reveals some space to refine capacity measurement at the point that existing general indicators cannot capture, but still, the structured capacity variation within the region largely explains health outcomes. Notwithstanding, Chaps. 6–8 suggest that the best response to the pandemic in terms of policy implementation and innovations might not necessarily be found in the state alone but in the interaction between the state and society. The state in cooperation with societal actors strives to respond although in ad hoc manner. Whether such instant solutions evolve into institutional upgrading awaits further studies.

Furthermore, some chapters of this volume disclose that the state is not a unitary entity. A key intra-governmental dynamic explored in this volume is the relationship between central and local governments. Chapter 2 reminds that Brazil's decentralized healthcare regime allowed local governments to act independently of the central government led by a populist president reluctant to implement COVID-19 measures. Looking more deeply, Chap. 5 reports that subnational disparities in Brazil's primary healthcare systems are path-dependent and have structured the uneven consequences (see also Schaefer et al., 2020).

Chapter 8 expands on this point by illustrating how collaborative governance involves not only central and local governments but also specialized public institutions (e.g., human rights commissions and public schools). These institutions, sometimes at odds with government leaders, played active roles in trying to facilitate citizen engagement in policy implementation. Likewise, Argentina's vaccine distribution process, characterized as a "patchwork" in Chap. 8, was not merely a straightforward allocation of resources by the central government. Instead, various actors within the government, such as the politically independent ANMAT (National Administration of Drugs, Food, and Medical Technology), engaged in trial and error while interacting with pharmaceutical companies and international organizations to establish an effective vaccine delivery system.

Reckoning with state weaknesses and state-society co-production suggests that what the state is capable of achieving does not hinge solely on the state but also on state–society interactions. This theoretical reconsideration goes beyond what state capacity, i.e., the capacity of the state, originally meant to be, which is worth considering in such a context where state capacity is weak but potentially complemented by other actors. We recognize that, when responding to the unknown threat of COVID-19, both government officials and ordinary citizens constantly deliberated on what measures would be best for society. In voluntary behavioral changes, like wearing masks or not, people take such precautions with or without the state announcement (Chap. 4). For the sake of a common goal that requires financial, technical, and accumulative contributions, the state and societal actors collaborate to fill the gap each side has (Chap. 8). These findings underscore the need to situate the discussion of state capacity within the context in which specific policy issues are unfolded. We should not be confused about what the state can do independently, but some policy targets need a broader viewpoint in the interaction with society.

9.5 Further Discussions and Limitations

Before closing this book, we highlight some additional messages regarding possible suggestions for future pandemics. What worked, how much it worked, and what could be done when it did not work are all useful knowledge for future challenges.

Moving beyond the long-term state-building, policy improvements under limited government resources necessitate cost-effective innovations. First, assessing policy effectiveness before implementation is crucial. One of the key findings of Chap. 4 discussing the mask-wearing announcements is that governments continued to encourage mask-wearing even when people were already sufficiently compliant. It is surprising that the so-called "ceiling effect," which is evident even for people without healthcare expertise, was often overlooked by policymakers. Second, technology may open new frontiers. As discussed in Chaps. 6 and 7, tools such as contact-tracing software, debit cards, and biometric authentication systems have enhanced efficiencies and amplified policy options. Given the rapid progress in information technology, future advancements are expected to further reduce costs and improve accessibility. Rather than viewing technological innovation as separate from public policy, it is essential to continually explore its everyday applications and build the necessary human networks (e.g., identifying relevant technical experts for consultation) to support its implementation. Such measures would significantly improve the efficiency of limited government resources.

The third consideration, closely related to the first two, involves compiling insights from COVID-19 responses and systematically organizing information to prepare for future pandemics. As repeatedly emphasized in this book, COVID-19 was a global crisis, turning the world into a laboratory for crisis response. Now that the pandemic has largely subsided, we possess a diverse range of experiences, along with numerous academic evaluations. For example, Chap. 3 developed an index for testing capacity, a significant contribution to measuring state capacity in a pandemic context. Systematically documenting such experiences and expertise—regardless of successes or failures—will help countries with low state capacity, particularly in Latin America, prepare for future health crises. Clarifying how many resources a government mobilized, whether they were effective, and what was lacking are important steps in guiding future budget allocations.

Enabling such efforts requires the government to make stable investments in human capital. Maintaining scientific and technological organizations within the government, as well as experts in public universities and research institutions, serves as a crucial societal safeguard. ANMAT, which played a central role in vaccine distribution and was featured in Chap. 8, exemplifies this point. Established in 1992 under Carlos Menem's neoliberal reforms in Argentina, ANMAT endured multiple political transitions and shifts between right-wing and left-wing administrations, yet its institutional continuity enabled it to play a pivotal role in the COVID-19 response. Furthermore, ensuring the retention of specialists in pandemic policy does not impose a significant financial burden. By maintaining a modest but dedicated group of professionals, governments can preserve institutional knowledge and ensure preparedness for future health crises without straining public resources.

In contrast to the three cost-effective strategies outlined above, cost-incurring measures directly address the challenges faced by Latin American governments and ultimately depend on policymakers' commitment. For example, the shortage of medical resources—such as hospital beds, doctors, and medicines—could be mitigated by consistently increasing public spending. However, this requires sustained agreement among politicians across ideological lines, as well as the reallocation of funds from other public services. As discussed in Chap. 7, collaborative governance allows for the efficient introduction of policies that integrate both governmental and non-governmental resources to meet citizens' needs. However, the realization of collaborative governance entails multiple challenges. To implement it effectively, policymakers must commit to initiatives without fear of failure, transcend partisan conflicts to establish cooperation, restore public trust in politics, and ensure transparent governance. Anyone engaged in Latin American politics understands that, despite the apparent necessity of these measures, their implementation is far from straightforward.

Last but not least, we acknowledge several thematic issues this collection does not address. An important structure or institution to be discussed is the political regime. As confirmed in the previous section, democracy—more specifically, constant elections—can induce risk-averse behavior among politicians. This negative evaluation might seem to support the argument favoring autocracy over democracy, which gained traction during the COVID-19 pandemic. However, this book does not adopt such a stance. First, among the findings established in this book, there are cases where democracy incentivizes politicians to adopt proactive policies. Chapter 7 presents an example from Chile, where a mayor who cooperated with citizens to implement COVID-19 measures was re-elected due to his demonstrated administrative competence. Second, recent research has not confirmed that autocratic regimes perform better in pandemic response (Annaka 2022; Martín-Martín et al. 2024). Third, regardless of pandemic performance, democracy itself holds inherent value and should be respected (Sen 1999). As noted in some previous studies and in Chap. 2 of this book, COVID-19 measures under autocratic regimes—or authoritarian decision-making within democratic regimes—undermine the principle of self-governance, where citizens freely express their opinions and decide on policies that govern them. Even as concerns over democratic backsliding persist, Latin American countries have experienced unprecedented continuity in democratic governance. Given this, democracy should be regarded as a given framework within which countermeasures should be considered.

Alongside political regimes, decentralization is also an institutional factor influencing government coordination and conflict. The evaluation of decentralization in this book is not clear-cut. As explained in the previous section, Chap. 2 showed that Brazil's decentralized healthcare regime functioned as a shelter for local governments against a populist president in decision-making related to counter-pandemic policies. However, at the same time, this chapter and Chap. 5 highlighted the importance of uniform service provision within a country when assessing healthcare quality, noting that COVID-19 exposed subnational disparities in healthcare services. This suggests the significance of the central government's role in addressing such inconsistencies. Moreover, Chap. 7, which discusses collaborative governance, identifies the conflict between central and local governments as an obstacle to cooperation. Based on these findings, a high degree of decentralization does not necessarily equate to an effective pandemic response.

Keeping these points in mind, the discussion of state capacity during the time of a pandemic enriches our understanding of what should be done for a better future. Ultimately, the effectiveness of the pandemic response in Latin America depends on the ability to navigate structural limitations, optimize institutional arrangements, and implement innovative policies tailored to local contexts. While challenges remain, the lessons drawn from COVID-19 highlight the importance of adaptive governance, long-term investment in institutional capacity, and a commitment to democratic principles. The future of public health preparedness in the region hinges on policymakers' ability to balance these factors while fostering resilience in the face of future crises.

References

Alfano, V., & Ercolano, S. (2022). Stay at home! Governance quality and effectiveness of lockdown. *Social Indicators Research, 159*(1), 101–123. https://doi.org/10.1007/s11205-021-02742-3

Annaka, S. (2022). Good democratic governance can combat COVID-19: Excess mortality analysis. *International Journal of Disaster Risk Reduction, 83*.

Bosancianu, C. M., Hilbig, H., Humphreys, M., Kc, S., Lieber, N., & Scacco, A. (2020). *Political and social correlates of Covid-19 mortality* [Preprint]. SocArXiv. https://doi.org/10.31235/osf.io/ub3zd

Brinks, D. M., Levitsky, S., & Murillo, M. V. (Eds.). (2020). *The politics of institutional weakness in Latin America*. Cambridge University Press.

Eaton, K. (2017). *Territory and ideology in Latin America: Policy conflicts between national and subnational governments*. Oxford University Press.

Gisselquist, R. M., & Vaccaro, A. (2023). COVID-19 and the state: Exploring a puzzling relationship in the early stages of the pandemic. *Journal of International Development, 35*(5), 800–819. https://doi.org/10.1002/jid.3702

Helmke, G., & Levitsky, S. (2004). Informal institutions and comparative politics: A research agenda. *Perspectives on Politics, 2*(4), 725–740.

Kurtz, M. J. (2013). *Latin American state building in comparative perspective: Social foundations of institutional order*. Cambridge University Press.

Martín-Martín, J. J., et al. (2024). Democratic quality and excess mortality during the COVID-19 pandemic. *Scientific Reports, 14*(1).

Saylor, R. (2014). *State building in boom times: Commodities and coalitions in Latin America and Africa*. Oxford University Press.

Schaefer, B. M., Resende, R. C., Epitácio, S. d. S. F., & Aleixo, M. T. (2020). Government actions against the new coronavirus: Evidence from the Brazilian states. *Revista de Administração Pública, 54*(5), 1429–1445. https://doi.org/10.1590/0034-761220200503x

Sen, A. (1999). *Development as freedom*. Oxford University Press.

Serikbayeva, B., Abdulla, K., & Oskenbayev, Y. (2021). State capacity in responding to COVID-19. *International Journal of Public Administration, 44*(11–12), 920–930. https://doi.org/10.1080/01900692.2020.1850778
Soifer, H. D. (2015). *State building in Latin America*. Cambridge University Press.
Yashar, D. J. (2018). *Homicidal ecologies: Illicit economies and complicit states in Latin America*. Cambridge University Press.

Index

I. Okada (ed.), *COVID-19 and State Capacity in Latin America*, Latin American Societies, https://doi.org/10.1007/978-3-032-15572-6

MIX
Papier aus verantwortungsvollen Quellen
Paper from responsible sources
FSC® C105338

FSC
www.fsc.org

If you have any concerns about our products,
you can contact us on
ProductSafety@springernature.com

In case Publisher is established outside the EU,
the EU authorized representative is:
Springer Nature Customer Service Center GmbH
Europaplatz 3, 69115 Heidelberg, Germany

Printed by Libri Plureos GmbH
in Hamburg, Germany